Carol

KU-062-283

current

nursing

practice

Accident and
Emergency Nursing

Current Nursing Practice titles

Accident and Emergency Nursing
Ear, Nose and Throat Nursing
Neuromedical and Neurosurgical Nursing
Plastic Surgical and Burns Nursing

Accident and Emergency Nursing

David Bradley, SRN, ONC (Hons)

Charge Nurse, Accident and Emergency Unit
Whiston Hospital, Prescot, Merseyside

Second edition

Baillière Tindall London Philadelphia Toronto
Mexico City Rio de Janeiro Sydney Tokyo Hong Kong

<u>Baillière Tindall</u> 1 St Anne's Road
W.B. Saunders Eastbourne, East Sussex BN21 3UN, England

West Washington Square
Philadelphia, PA 19105, USA

1 Goldthorne Avenue
Toronto, Ontario M8Z 5T9, Canada

Apartado 26370 — Cedro 512
Mexico 4, DF Mexico

Rua Evaristo da Veiga 55, 20° andar
Rio de Janeiro — RJ, Brazil

ABP Australia Ltd, 44–50 Waterloo Road
North Ryde, NSW 2113, Australia

Ichibancho Central Building, 22–1 Ichibancho
Chiyoda-Ku, Tokyo 102, Japan

10/fl, Inter-Continental Plaza, 94 Granville Road
Tsim Sha Tsui East, Kowloon, Hong Kong

© 1984 Baillière Tindall. All rights reserved. No part of this publication
may be reproduced, stored in a retrieval system or transmitted,
in any form or by any means, electronic, mechanical, photocopying
or otherwise, without the prior permission of Baillière Tindall,
1 St Anne's Road, Eastbourne, East Sussex BN21 3UN, England

First published as Nurses' Aids Series Special Interest Text 1980
Reprinted 1982
Second edition 1984

Typeset by Photo-Graphics, Honiton, Devon
Printed and bound in Great Britian by
William Clowes Ltd, Beccles and London

British Library Cataloguing in Publication Data

Bradley, David, 1945–
  Accident and emergency nursing.—2nd ed.
  —(Current nursing practice)
  1. Emergency nursing
  I. Title II. Series
  610.73′61   RT120.E4

ISBN 0–7020–1048–0

Contents

Preface

Accident and emergency nursing, although a vital and growing specialty, has little specific nursing literature with which to form even a backbone of knowledge. Because of this, teaching is made more difficult, standards vary and we are carried along by the enthusiasm and literature written by our medical staff. I have long felt that this is a truly damning fact against our branch of the profession. The aim of my book is, therefore, to start to fill this enormous gap in nursing literature.

It must now be fully realized that accident and emergency nursing is a specialty with its own body of knowledge, not merely a branch of orthopaedics or a miscellany of conditions which other specialties do not want. The use of ward attitudes and theory is no longer good enough. New priorities have to be used, patients with problems outside accidents and emergencies must be refused care, non-urgent admissions must pass straight through, dressings must be done a different way: the list is endless. Then and only then can we realize our primary objective, to become masters of resuscitation and the immediate care of accidents and emergencies.

The realms of medical and nursing knowledge are closely intertwined and will always be so because both deal with patients. I have, however, done my best to provide as pure a book of nursing as I can. In these times accident and emergency specialist nurses in emergency situations must be proficient at intubation, setting up intravenous infusions, defibrillation and other tasks, otherwise patients will simply die. But in addition to this, nurses must also retain their old tasks of talking to and caring about people, of applying the splint or cleaning the wound, otherwise they will no longer be nurses.

I have chosen the subjects of the chapters with great care, trying to place myself in the 'shoes' of both learners and trained nurses who are to start work on accident and emergency units. The book contains most of the information which each will require to become an effective team member. Starting with essential preliminaries of proficiency in dealing with extreme emergencies, I have progressed through the moderately severe injuries of orthopaedic trauma to the more minor problems encountered in our everyday life, for example nose bleeds and drunks.

The book more than covers nursing aspects of the ENB syllabus for accident and emergency nursing (Courses 198 and 201), and should be of immense help to all trained nurses who cannot attend such a course locally. For learners it will serve as a substantial reference book while they work on the unit and should also help them with resuscitation throughout their lives. Nurses involved in pure orthopaedics, especially those taking the ONC course, will find much that is of use to them, as will nurses working on ITUs, giving all a firm grounding in trauma nursing. I would also like to think that it will gain some readers among our friends in the ambulance service. Apart from helping them to appreciate some of our problems, most of the chapters contain something to interest them.

No one part of the book should be read in complete isolation, for to do so would give an incomplete picture of patients and their priorities. With the present medical structure of many accident and emergency units, one frequently works with casualty officers who may lack experience in accident work and have either no specialist registrar back-up or a slow back-up. In such circumstances with a critically ill patient by the time he or she is seen, first by the casualty officer, then by the registrar and finally by a consultant, it is too late. The experienced accident and emergency nurse must be able to help fill this gap, becoming the right hand and often the guiding hand of the doctor. It is a senior nurse's moral and legal responsibility to ensure that no harm comes to the patient; never is this more acutely felt than in an emergency. This book aims to give you the knowledge for correct decision making while your day-to-day experience slowly accumulates.

In this second edition the whole of the book has been thoroughly revised and updated, and many illustrations have been added or replaced. This was found to be necessary both to keep up-to-date with this fast-changing specialty and in response to suggestions for improvement from many sources worldwide.

New chapters will be found on such subjects as paediatric problems, care of the elderly and the aggressive patient. There are also many new sections, for instance, the nursing process, emergency childbirth and flying squads.

I hope that this new edition will meet most of your needs. Please write and let me know if you have any comments. It is only by hearing such suggestions that it can remain the accident and emergency nurse's first choice.

David Bradley

Acknowledgements

My thanks go mainly to my wife Brenda; I owe her a great deal for her suffering as she deciphered my notorious handwriting, for making countless corrections and for typing my manuscript in both editions. Next in line comes Mr Ron Brislen who, during the preparation of the first edition, spent many hours helping me with suggestions and illustrations, correcting technicalities in the manuscript and giving constructive criticism. Since his tragic death in 1982 I have 'gone it alone' but much of the flavour of the book still reflects his enthusiasm and thoughts. I also thank Miss McNally and all the staff of the Accident and Emergency Unit at Whiston Hospital, who have given me so many excellent nursing ideas over the years; this book is very much what they strive to achieve.

Mr S. Bailey of the Cheshire ambulance service helped me in the writing of the section about the ambulance service and its equipment in the first edition, and since then both he and his colleagues in the Cheshire and Merseyside ambulance services have kept me well informed of improvements, for which I thank them.

For doing so much of the modelling for the photographs, without any complaint, I wish to thank my two sons, Stephen and Paul — they were invaluable.

I wish to thank a nursing colleague, Miss Ada Masterton, for contributing many new illustrations to the book. Her artistic skill has brought to life much of my text and given me a means of expressing my ideas. I only hope that, as the years go by, more of the illustrations can be converted to her style.

For help with the section on head injuries I wish to thank Miss Olga Ferdinand from the Department of Neurology, Walton Hospital, and also Dr Trevor Smith of the same department for information about CAT scans.

The firms which have helped me with information and photographs are: 3M (UK) Ltd; F. W. Equipment Co. Ltd; Capecraft Ltd; Medic-Alert Foundation; Seton Products Ltd; Ambu International; Loxley Medical; J.O.B.S.T. Institute; Ciba Geigy.

Last, but by no means least, I wish to thank the staff of Baillière Tindall for all their guidance and encouragement.

To my wife Brenda

1 An introduction to the accident and emergency department

How can you explain to a newcomer what working in an accident and emergency department is like, when there is no such thing as a typical working day? The department's mood can change by the minute, snatching you from playing games with a young child, to the tension of major trauma and back again to conversation with an elderly frightened lady literally within minutes. Suffice it to say because of the tremendous variety of work every learner will find at worst a few aspects which will be of interest to them and at best their experience on the department will be the most exhilarating of their whole career.

Many nurses, trained and untrained alike, have an abject fear of the mere thought of accident and emergency work. In most instances this is because they have a vision of being left alone to cope with some diabolical emergency. The truth is far from this; you will be introduced gradually to responsibility, helping in simple ways when a serious emergency arrives. Then, as your confidence and familiarity increase so will your responsibility and involvement with the critically ill.

The intention of this book is to give both learners and trained staff an insight into the world of 'accident and emergency' and how to cope with the nursing of the majority of conditions which they will face.

FUNCTIONS OF THE DEPARTMENT

Let us now consider what the aims and functions of an accident and emergency department should be:

- Perhaps the most obvious function of all is that we must always be ready to care for the severely injured or ill at any time of the day or night even if we are already busy. But look carefully at my words 'at any time of the day or night'. This means that the staff on duty at 3 a.m. must be just as highly qualified as those on duty between 9 a.m. and 5 p.m., and must be of adequate number too. Similarly, 'even if we are already busy', means that we must always have an eye to what may come in. We should never have all the resuscitation bays full, and resuscitation equipment should always be completely ready for use.

- Next in line comes the caring of the myriad of everyday trauma such as fractures, burns, lacerations, sprains, etc. Although I have placed this group of injuries second on my list, it forms the greater part of our work, that is, our 'bread and butter'.
- In some hospitals the accident and emergency department is also used as an admission unit, GPs sending patients in for assessment with a view to admission. Such a state is a tremendous added burden and must be taken account of when thinking of available space and staff. An admission unit must never drain or block the resources available for resuscitation. Departments with and without such facilities will require very different staffing and floor space.
- To be an ever-open door, a safety valve, where help and advice can be gained by any member of the public in distress when they have nowhere else to turn. An example of this group would be a new arrival in a district who becomes ill and does not have a GP.
- To make contingency plans for action in a major incident and to provide an accident flying squad.
- To care for the relatives of patients who are brought in dead.
- To provide follow up by way of clinic facilities for the review of injured patients.
- To provide certain surgical facilities. This depends on the hospital and can vary from incision of abscesses and removal of small foreign bodies and cysts to comparatively major surgical procedures (e.g. the opening of a chest or abdomen or the making of burr holes).

Sadly, however, the service is much abused. It is becoming increasingly common to see the departments used as a GP service by patients often too lazy to go to see their own doctors. GPs themselves are not blameless, some simply sending any problem to their local accident and emergency department as an easy way out. This problem is highlighted at night, at week-ends and at Bank Holidays when adequate outside help is hard to obtain.

At present the accident and emergency service in this country is still in a state of change. The best is very, very good, the worst I have experienced is quite inadequate and the remainder, which includes most of us, lie somewhere in between. Too often, whether a patient lives or dies following critical injury depends on where the incident occurred or at what time of day it occurred, whereas every patient no matter how humble should have the most excellent care. If the care that we give our patients can be improved on in any other unit then we are not giving them the care they deserve. There is no shame in being equalled, only in being less than the best.

However, the accident and emergency department is not the only determinant of the patient's survival. We are just one link in a long chain of care which starts at the roadside and continues until the patient is rehabilitated into normal life. It only requires one of these links to be non-existent or inefficient for the patient to perish, be permanently maimed or suffer considerable pain. For us to be able to operate to best effect we must know and closely liaise with the other nearby links. To give an example of this, involving oneself with the training of the general public in First Aid will 'spread the gospel' of resuscitation and so help to lessen the shameful number of unnecessary deaths which would be prevented, for instance, by simple clearing of the airway. Also, frequent meetings with the ambulance service help each side to understand the other's problems, to increase their knowledge and to realize the other's difficulties and limitations.

NURSE EDUCATION

Teaching is not the job of one or two senior people on the department, rather it should be the combined efforts of all staff to make a 'learning environment'. In this way every patient and every treatment becomes a learning opportunity. Time and help need to be given to all the grades of trained staff for this sadly alien role.

The very nature of accident and emergency work means that there is seldom time available to explain something for more than 15 minutes at a time without interruption. It is, however, important that a system is worked out so that small tutorials do occur at regular intervals, both to discuss cases which have been through the department and to follow a simple programme of essential subjects and procedures. Trained staff too should meet regularly during or after work to keep abreast of the times and keep up interest in accident and emergency subjects. A group evaluation of our effectiveness during resuscitation and further care of a trauma victim is essential, highlighting our good and bad points to help both staff and future trauma victims. The more junior trained staff can present interesting cases to the group from time to time, while the senior ones can lecture on a given subject.

Learners must know what is expected of them during their accident and emergency experience, just as all the trained staff must know what to show or teach. Clear objectives must therefore be laid down so that all can see the path ahead.

Learning opportunities will vary between departments but the nurse should take the opportunity:

- To discuss the role of the accident and emergency service as a whole.
- To discover the functions of the accident and emergency department.
- To understand the role of the ambulance service and its difficulties.
- To learn how to maintain and operate emergency equipment, and to have it ready for immediate use.
- To be able to resuscitate a critical patient, i.e. to perform ECM, artificial ventilation, airway clearance and stop haemorrhage, and to assist the doctor with intubation, setting up i.v.s and chest drains, and defibrillation.
- To understand the actions and problems associated with the following drugs: ATT, Humotet, penicillin and other antibiotics, morphine and its derivatives, adrenaline, ipecacuanha, sodium bicarbonate, calcium and paracetamol.
- To be able to assess the seriousness of a patient's condition (the elements of triage).
- To be able to receive a patient, put them at ease, assess their problems, care for their property and talk to their relatives.
- To prepare patients for the doctor's examination.
- To efficiently observe patients with common conditions and record the findings (e.g. head injuries and chest pains).
- To know about and be able to help with care and treatment of patients with common injuries and emergency conditions (e.g.

overdoses, fractured femur, Colles' fracture, haemorrhage, chest pains, cardiac arrest and head injuries.

- To be able to assess a patient's needs on discharge.
- To be competent at simple treatments (e.g. crêpe bandages, splints, Steristrips, and wound and burn dressings.
- To be able to assist with the following: stomach washouts, Thomas splints and sutures.
- To understand the role of people associated with the accident and emergency department (i.e Community Nurses, Health Visitors, Police, Press, Clergy).
- To know of the practical problems associated with the death of a patient and to be able to help with the care of the relatives.
- To understand the special needs of children in the Department and to be alert to the problems of non-accidental injury (NAI).
- To know of and understand our Flying Squad role.
- To become efficient in the practice of the first-aid treatments.

All learners should have a list both of their objectives and of the various procedures which they should carry out or see in action during the period spent in the department so that they have a rough measure of their progress.

With the above 'plan' in operation all levels of staff benefit from the teaching environment which will prevail. The next stage of learning is the questioning of what has been taught previously. This is a lead up to research and it is through research that we as a profession can develop. Research requires careful planning and knowledge, but groups are available in different regions to help with this and to finance projects. Below are a few simple clinical nursing subjects in the accident and emergency field which could benefit from nursing research:

- Stomach washout, method and effectiveness
- Use of clean gloves for dressings
- The comparative efficiency of various supporting bandages
- The use of the new skin 'glue'
- The most efficient layout of equipment in a resuscitation area

THE NURSING PROCESS

Over recent years much has been written about the nursing process in general, but scarcely anything about its application in the accident and emergency department. So, let us have some general thoughts on the matter. Firstly, let us understand that there is no place at all in a busy accident and emergency department for the formal writing of nursing care plans as seen on the wards. Secondly, an emergency situation is a situation of practised routines of action. Any history, plan, implementation and assessment is done instantaneously and the necessary notes are made afterwards. But, in training nurses for emergency care, the nursing process sets out a reasonable method of training your mind to think systematically about the care required.

So how, you may ask, do we set about using the nursing process in accident and emergency departments? The secret is in being adaptable. When patients are admitted to wards they are usually in for a reasonable length of time, and therefore a full assessment can be made of their needs, a care plan implemented and as time goes by the success or failure of the plan can be evaluated. This contrasts sharply with an accident and emergency department where our patient will be with us for a matter of only minutes to a maximum of several hours. Full assessment and follow ups are out of the question, but we can go some way towards the process; a way which is realistic and blends in with the time available. You see, this is not too far from the original idea. The nursing process is *not* paperwork, writing reports and filling in forms. The nursing process is talking to patients, finding out their problems, deciding what you can do to help, getting on with the job and making sure it is working *plus* writing a note so that others know what is to be done. On an accident and emergency unit what we have to do is implement a logical and systematic approach to patient care with the minimum of extra writing and paperwork.

The nursing process used with minor injuries

The majority of the work load on an accident and emergency department is concerned with what to us are comparatively minor injuries. Let me now give an example of how the nursing process can be adapted to the requirements of this type of patient. Suppose that you are looking after a patient with a sprained ankle. In the two or three minutes while you are bandaging the ankle it should already be second nature to talk to the patient, finding out how and why the accident happened. Depending on his physical state, age, etc. you may have to ask how he will be able to cope at home or whether the injury will affect his job, sport or finances. In the majority of cases no problems will arise and we can sign to this effect when we complete the treatment. However, if while talking to the patient a problem surfaces which is within our sphere we can make a very brief note about it.

From my visits to other departments, most seem to have adequate space on the reverse side of the patients' case papers or cards to enable nursing comments to be written without the need for separate sheets of paper. Separate sheets of paper should be avoided if possible since it means extra writing, *implies* much extra work for nurses, and can get lost or will be folded away out of sight and not used. Extra paper is a psychological barrier to be avoided.

So, we simply have a small rubber stamp on the back of our patient's card as shown in Fig. 1. On this we write the patient's problem or problems and what we have done. For example, our patient with a sprained ankle could have eczema of the underlying skin requiring daily applications of creams, or difficulty in walking unaided, or a social problem such as having to attend an exam. All items like these can be mentioned as shown in Fig. 2A. At the next visit while the nurse is treating the patient, she can enquire how the nursing actions have affected the problems and once again make a very *brief* note (Fig. 2B). All the way along the line it must be stressed that there is no sitting down and purposefully question-

Problem	Action	Outcome

Fig. 1. *The layout for nursing notes.*

A

Problem	Action	Outcome
16/7 Eczema at ankle, on daily Betnovate	Nurse visit daily → cream + bandage	
Difficulty in weight bearing	Try stick	
'A' level is on 27th	Private sick note Bring next appt. forward	

B

Problem	Action	Outcome
16/7 Eczema at ankle, on daily Betnovate	Nurse visit daily → cream + bandage	21/7 Eczema satisfactory, continue with nurse
Difficulty in weight bearing	Try stick	✓
'A' level is on 27th	Private sick note Bring next appt. forward	Is taking exam

Fig. 2. A and B. *The filling in of the notes.*

ing the patient. There is only time for simple, everyday, friendly conversation which will actually uncover problems far more easily and also let the patient know that you have a genuine interest in him. A good 70 to 80 per cent of this type of patient will not have any problems requiring action or referral.

The nursing process used with serious injuries

A similar approach can be used for patients with more serious injuries who are to be admitted to the wards. But, it must be a simple extension of what we already do and then only if the time is available; even brief notes should not interfere with our routine emergency care. As an example now, let us consider a patient with a fractured shaft of femur following a road traffic accident (RTA), who is shortly to be sent to the ward.

All our usual care has been carried out, the patient's condition is stable, his leg is splinted and he has had adequate analgesia. Such a time is bad for any but the most important of questions, but items like those shown in Fig. 3 can easily come to light, are easily noted down quickly and will help the ward staff to care for the patient more efficiently.

Problem	Action	Outcome
1. Patient's mother still not contacted	Clerk to inform	/
2. Graze (L) buttock @ ring of splint	Cleaned + dressed	/
3. Patient doesn't know A.T.T. status	Ward to ask parents later	/
4. Circulation and sensation in leg	Observation of Dorsalis pedis, toe sensation + movements	OK on leaving A + E

Fig. 3. *The notes used for seriously injured patients.*

The nursing process used for elderly infirm patients who are to go home

Finally, another method is best used when dealing with elderly infirm patients. This involves the use of a detailed check list which at a push could be rubber stamped onto the back of an existing card but would probably have to go on a separate sheet (Fig. 4). A similar system has been in use at Whiston Hospital for many years and has proved to be quite workable. The most important point about this form is that although it is comparatively quick to fill in, it still takes up to ten minutes to fill in even for an experienced

NAME:	DATE:
ASSESSMENT	
Lives with: Self, Husband, Relatives	
Accommodation: House, Flat	
Bed: Upstairs, Downstairs	
Toilet: Upstairs, Commode, Bed pan, Bottle, etc.	
Food:	
Mobility: Before After	
Shopping:	
Heating:	
Physical state: Clean, Dirty, Good, Poor	
Hearing: **Vision:** **Appliances:**	
Mental state: Sensible, Confused	
Services: Home Help District Nurse Health Visitor Social Services Meals on Wheels Relatives Friends Neighbours	
Pets: **Keys:** **Valuables:**	
Accident detail:	
Nurse	

Fig. 4. *An assessment form used for elderly patients.*

trained nurse. Before elderly patients are sent home it is essential for us to be sure that they can cope, and the only way to do this is to gain a full idea of their background and abilities. The one point on our side is that the time element is flexible, i.e. if necessary an emergency can be coped with until a nurse is free to spend time getting to know the patient. Any form which involves much writing is totally unacceptable in an accident and emergency unit.

THE DESIGN OF ACCIDENT AND EMERGENCY UNITS

Design is not directly a nurse's job, but a unit built without the prior advice of a nurse will have many failings, often of major importance. Specialist accident and emergency nurses should be involved in the earliest consultations with the architect. They should also be involved regularly during the whole planning and building operation. Those chosen for this task must have the ability to read a plan correctly and have enough insight into the day-to-day running of the unit to forsee what problems a given layout will cause.

A few thoughts on design:

- An easily accessible entrance with space for several ambulances at a time, plus ample turning space.
- Separate entrances for stretcher cases and walking wounded.
- A resuscitation bay adjacent to the main entrance.
- Even if the unit is part of a general hospital, suitable space should be provided for children and should be decorated accordingly.
- The reception office should be centrally placed because everything revolves around it. Nurses should have the minimum of walking to find documents.
- The majority of cubicles should not have doors; patients can die behind closed doors and not be noticed.
- The resuscitation area should be larger than you might at first imagine. Those who have never seen the reception of a critically injured patient will find it hard to believe how much floor space is required for comfort. The resuscitation area should be capable of dealing with at least two critically injured people.
- A quiet room should be available for the relatives of deceased patients. This room must not be too far away from the working area.

- A staff rest room where you can relax and unwind for a few minutes, if necessary. However, this often tends to get pushed into the background if finance is short.
- Ample space should be available to position large toys in the waiting areas to keep children occupied.
- Sister's office should be within viewing distance of the resuscitation bay.
- X-ray facilities should be available in the department, or at least nearby.
- Everything should be on one level with easy access for wheelchairs to the toilets, etc.
- Ample shelving so that emergency items are on display.
- Stores near to the 'action' so that 'topping up' is not tiresome.

SOME ASPECTS OF ACCIDENT AND EMERGENCY MANAGEMENT

Although its effects are not as immediate, ineffectual organization, management and lack of teaching will kill your patient just as surely as poor resuscitation. No one person can make an accident service good or bad; it is the cumulative result of team work. The heads of both medical and nursing services can, however, have a profound effect on what occurs and by their very attitude to the job and staff make the department a place either of excellence, happiness, enthusiasm and learning or on the other hand of frustration, monotony and stagnation. The staff of an accident and emergency unit are its most valuable commodity. Miracles can be performed in poor conditions with antiquated equipment if only the staff have a combination of enthusiasm and knowledge.

A major factor affecting nursing staff on accident and emergency units is stress. I will go further to state that there are few places in the hospital service where the level of nursing stress is so intense as on an accident and emergency unit. I list my reasons below:

1. Literally any disease or injury imaginable can come through the emergency doors at any time without notice.
2. If a ward is full it can accept no more; if an accident and emergency department is full it must continue accepting patients and still remain capable of responding to any emergency.

3. The specialist accident and emergency nurse has to be able to cope with the above, occasionally for several minutes without the assistance of a doctor.
4. The situation also occurs when the nurse is the most experienced person on the scene, working with very junior and inexperienced medical staff.
5. Death is an everyday occurrence, often in the most tragic of circumstances and 'out of the blue'.
6. Violence which is seldom seen on the wards can occur with regularity. Aggression is also seen more frequently from both relatives and patients.

A formidable list, and one which can be added to.

Qualities

I am frequently asked 'What are the qualities of a good accident and emergency nurse?' In choosing staff for the unit bear in mind the previously mentioned list and try to decide if the nurse will be able to cope with the situations which will surely present themselves at some time. Proficiency, or at least an interest, in resuscitation is a very basic need, plus the ability to adapt quickly to changing circumstances. Panic is deadly on the unit and spreads like fire; it must be avoided at all cost. Nurses showing this tendency must be removed, both for their own good and for that of the patients, unless the problem can be overcome with strict guidance. The nurse must be able to take command of a situation quickly and act decisively. Before being left in charge of a unit the nurse must have had an adequate training plus experience under supervision. Training should consist ideally of the JBCNS course or, where none is available locally, working on a unit while intensively studying all allied fields with the help of unit sisters. When first left in charge, a nurse needs expert accident and emergency nursing back-up to be available at the end of a telephone, just in case problems outside her experience crop up. A further feeling of security will prevail if there is an active, enthusiastic and knowledgeable medical presence. Other qualities are those generally expected of a nurse, for instance, kindness and compassion for others: without these you may as well call yourself a technician. Lastly, but by no means least, I must mention a sense of humour since without this you will be a very trying person to have around when we are all under stress. I go as far as to warn students of this in their pre-accident and emergency study block so that they understand why they may sometimes see trained staff laughing and joking about some tragedy which has just occurred. You need to laugh to stop yourself crying!

Staffing

Much could be said about staffing levels, but one basic point is that if the department is a major accident unit, an *experienced* sister should be present 24 hours a day. It is only with this expertise and experience that a totally efficient service can be provided. To fail to provide this minimum of care results in added suffering for the patient and the occasional death! Failure to provide this minimum level of care must surely be termed negligence.

This leaves us with the problem of staff nurses or enrolled nurses taking charge of the department. It is my opinion that this should only occur at times of crisis, for example sickness or staff leaving. Not that the nurse will not be able to cope—99 per cent of the time! It is the other 1 per cent which worries me, the problem which will only be seen occasionally: Münchausen's syndrome, atypical coronary thrombosis, extradural haemorrhage, a battered child or an unstable cervical fracture. Will the nurse be able to guide the doctor inexperienced in casualty to make correct decisions? The public subconsciously expects and definitely deserves this level of experience to be there when it is required.

Minimum staffing levels required to care effectively for various emergency conditions can be worked out with thought and a little research. I have calculated that four nurses is the minimum for a cardiac arrest or a major injury victim. Details of this can be found in an article in *A & E News* (see list of **Further reading** at the end of the chapter).

Readiness

The boy scouts' motto 'be prepared' could very well apply equally to accident and emergency departments. Never is a department in a more vulnerable position than when it already has one dire emergency or has just cleared one and the resuscitation area is completely disorganized. This needs to be pointed out because being busy with one emergency is no insurance that another is not already occurring.

I always believe that the best type of accident and emergency unit is an empty one. I do not, however, mean by this that patients should be 'hurried through' but neither do I feel that patients should stay in the department a minute longer than is necessary. I would love to delay some of the most technically interesting injuries but know this is impossible. But similarly, the patients who 'no one wants' must also go so that our prime function is not endangered. General hospital staff throughout the country seem to think that, because there is plenty of room available in an accident and emergency department, it is there for general use, be it for clerking patients or waiting an hour for another opinion. It is rare indeed that someone who does not work on an accident and emergency department realizes how rapidly scenes can change from tranquillity to storm and how valuable an extra nurse or an extra cubicle can be.

The work load

The number of patients which a ward deals with in a day is to some extent controllable. Accident and emergency departments start off with an obviously uncontrollable number of new patients. But a great deal of the burden of responsibility for excessive work loads must be on the shoulders of the doctors. Although many are first-rate at forcing patients to get treatment through the correct channels, many give in to the patients' whims and run what is in many instances a general practice or polyclinic, even following cases through two or three times instead of referring them. This situation is more common with doctors who are trained in other countries and are unfamiliar with the real purpose of an accident and emergency unit when they first arrive in the UK.

Another common mistake is the idea that conditions will heal in set man-made times. The prime example of this is the patient asked to return for review in 'a week', instead of serious thought being given to the number of days in which a condition will either heal or require more attention. This is just another way of giving yourself more work unnecessarily, not to mention the inconvenience to the patient.

Lastly, depending on the prevailing local system, many patients are asked to return to the department (for example, suture removal and dressings) when our community colleagues would be only too happy to take on some of the burden.

To change patients' attitudes is an uphill battle all the way but it is well worth while when it rewards you by giving you more time to perform your correct function.

THOUGHTS ON PLANNING FOR A MAJOR DISASTER

From an accident and emergency nurse's point of view a 'major disaster' is not a state which suddenly exists only after a specific number of casualties are expected. It is relative to the number and quality of staff available, the size of the department, the equipment available, the location of other hospitals nearby and other factors. An 'all-or-nothing' response is not the ideal answer. For example, 20 moderately injured casualties at one hospital will require only some of the staff on call to help in the department and some of those in the x-ray department and theatre to be alerted but not all. Some form of staged response must be formulated.

Perhaps the single most important decision to be made is whether a major incident has occurred and thus whether the machinery requires setting into motion. A senior hospital person must make this decision. What is major to police, fire and even ambulance staff is not necessarily major to the accident and emergency unit.

In any 'disaster' the patients must be categorized:

1. The shaken up
2. The 'walking wounded': those who have comparatively trivial injuries, for instance, a fractured humerus or lacerations
3. The serious stretcher case, for instance, the patient with a fractured femur who will easily be able to make it to hospital and is fully expected to live
4. The critical patient, for example, the unconscious patient with a head injury, a flail chest or severe shock
5. The dead

As a general rule it is not advantageous for the receiving hospital to send out a team to the site of the incident, although such a decision must be a local one taking into account the district and the facilities available.

Action at the site

Action at the site of a disaster must differ from that at a standard 'flying squad' attendance. In one situation you have many people looking after mainly one person, whereas in a disaster, care by a few has to be rationed out to the many depending on their needs. Perhaps the most vital job of all at the scene of the disaster is the division of patients into the five categories listed previously and the channelling of the teams to those who need them most. Too much time spent on a patient in the wrong category results in the death of others.

At the site, care will usually consist of airway care and volume replacement plus occasional surgery for a trapped patient (i.e. 'suck out, pump in and pack').

Depending on the types of disaster, different numbers of patients will leave the scene at different stages. The supreme example of this is to compare the staggered flow of patients at the Moorgate tube crash in London due to poor access for rescue staff, to the situation found at the London bomb blasts where access to the injured presented few problems and the flow of patients was rapid. The first patients to leave the site may not be the most seriously hurt. While speaking to the men of the Belfast ambulance service, one of the points which stuck firmly in my mind was that, when they first arrive on the scene of a bomb blast, the more trivially wounded tended to walk or be taken to the ambulance and so fill it up before the seriously injured were reached. Passers-by also pick up the more trivially injured in cars and take them directly to hospital.

If the equipment used is kept to one side, never used and rarely seen, it is unfair to expect staff to work efficiently with it under stress conditions. Any medical equipment which is used should be based on the existing 'flying squad' equipment with which everyone has a reasonable level of familiarity. Any boxes or packs should be identical, there being simply an increase in the number of sets available.

Hospital preparations

The allocation of tasks for the incident is something which will have to be discussed by many disciplines. However, at unit level it is fairly straight-forward.

It should never be presumed that the incident will occur at 10 a.m. on a Monday in May when everyone is available. Always have in your mind midnight on a Friday in mid-August. A staff nurse is in charge of the unit because the night sister is off sick; there is one other nurse on duty, a student. The unit is fairly busy with drunks and road traffic accidents. The nursing officer is away on holiday and the accident and emergency consultant is having a night out. Add to this a little rain and we are all prepared!

It is incorrect to start preparing equipment immediately. Your first duty is to get some extra pairs of hands for the expected deluge. This will involve getting someone on the phone, using an entirely up-to-date list which contains not only the private phone numbers of the staff, but also of one or two other places where they might be if out, for example, parents or friends. This job can become elaborate and should be delegated to a clerk as soon as possible. Volunteer helpers who do not know the unit well are only of very limited use and will require 'waiting on' or will have to be given more trivial tasks than they would usually do.

Clear all walking wounded from the department; they must either wait to be seen, perhaps for many hours, or simply go home and return later. Of the remaining patients, some must be warded immediately to make trolleys and bays available. Other review areas attached to the main accident and emergency unit will have to be opened up and you must still expect to have some quite serious injuries in them. All the critical patients, however, should be kept in or near the usual resuscitation area.

Staff, your most valuable commodity, have been sought. So has space in which to place your wounded. Next stock up the cubicles and treatment areas with all necessary emergency equipment.

The most senior nurse must remain mobile at all times, lending the occasional hand but staying basically free. Her task is to integrate the work of *everyone* so that they all know what they are to do.

Only category three or four patients should come to the accident and emergency unit. All others should go to another predetermined part of the hospital, for example, clinics. It can be a literally fatal mistake for a category one or two patient to 'block' a resuscitation cubicle.

Documentation will be a major headache. Identification by tagging must be done on arrival at the door, with both a number and a name if available. A central register of patients must be kept for enquiries and some form of emergency case sheet must be made up within minutes. You therefore have:

1. A labelled patient
2. A case sheet
3. A central list

Do not assume that the junior doctors will be able to organize by themselves. Often, casualty officers are 'passers by', coming perhaps only six months after they join the hospital staff; they cannot be expected to know all the schemes available. Also locums are commonly in use and doctors whose native tongue is not English may as a result be encountering organizational difficulties. Help as best you can.

MEDICOLEGAL PITFALLS AND COMPLAINTS

To understand medicolegal problems and complaints we must compare our situation with that on a ward. These problems abound on an accident and emergency unit. If we are nursing someone on a ward we build up a relationship during the patient's stay. The patient becomes familiar with our routines and to some extent understands our problems. Similarly, we find out what type of person the patient is and we can therefore handle the situation better. On an accident and emergency unit this cannot occur: 90 per cent of our patients are strangers and we see so little of them that we cannot judge easily how they will react to anything we say or do. The patient does not know any of our routines and problems. Most complaints are made because the person genuinely feels that he has been wronged. In my own experience a high proportion of complaints are caused by the patient or relative having a lack of information or a misunderstanding about what has occurred. This type of complaint is fairly easily cleared up at the time with tact and understanding. I give as an example patients who have to wait a long time before being treated (a major source of stress for both patients and nurses). Here a few words of explanation can make all the difference. If the complaint is valid, the breakdown in communication must be identified and remedied. Missing property is another perennial problem which can cause bitterness, suspicion, worry and paperwork. The only watertight answer is written evidence and witnesses and this just does not tie in well with the emergency situation. Human life must always come before property, but in the accident and emergency unit the patient's property must always come a close second if we are to do our jobs efficiently. Even a lack of valuables must be noted. Accusations of nursing negligence in one form or another occur occasionally, but are far less frequent than the problems mentioned above.

Problems occur when the treatment which the nurse has given varies from what the doctor has written on the patient's card. Such problems can be very subtle and because of this the investigation of the complaint will probably be led by a nursing manager.

Advice over the phone can be another tricky business, leading the unwary into trouble. Simply saying 'we cannot give advice over the phone' and leaving it at that is too off-hand and will offend many. After all, they require assistance and that is what we are all here for. A short non-committal (yet helpful) conversation is best, explaining to some extent what options they have open to them. Never give positive yes or no answers to questions which only the doctor can answer legally. A lot of trouble can result. You should be extremely wary of giving outsiders information about patients' conditions or their names and addresses, especially over the phone. Often the problem can be overcome simply by asking the patient if it is all right to inform the person making the enquiries. Even the police are only ordinarily entitled to medical details from a patient's notes if the patient has given permission. Nonetheless, you should also do your best to answer questions and help the police officer with brief details. The police will be invaluable to you, especially following road accidents, finding out who patients are and how accidents occurred, and contacting next of kin. A reasonable level of patient information should be readily available to the traffic police, even without the patient's consent. They have a right to know a vague diagnosis and some personal details. The specialist accident and emergency nurse should also be experienced enough to decide whether the traffic police should be allowed to talk to the patient.

Legalities of emergency procedures

The legal aspects of certain procedures could well be clarified here. I refer firstly, to the following treatments which are included in the appendix (i.e. endotracheal intubation, venepuncture, emergency laryngostomy).

Some call them 'non-nursing duties', but I consider that to be the case only if a doctor is immediately available. What we must remember is that some senior accident and emergency nurses are frequently on their own in some departments, often for many minutes before the arrival of medical assistance, and even then that medical assistance may be very inexperienced. In such situations the above procedures become essential nursing duties.

But that is not the end of the story I'm afraid, because in many (and I suspect most) accident and emergency departments in this country, you will *not* be legally covered by your Divisional Health Authority (DHA) to perform such emergency procedures even if you consider it life-saving, unless of course the consultant in charge of the department will take full responsibility for you.

So, let us assume that you attempt to intubate a patient, things go wrong and you put the tube into the oesophagus by mistake, a relative hears about it and threatens legal action. Unless your consultant is prepared to take the responsibility, you are in trouble.

We therefore have a situation in which if we sit back and let the patient die while we wait for a doctor or a senior doctor, then *we have no worries* about the legality of the situation because we have done all that is expected of an ordinary nurse. If, however, we bravely try to do, for instance, an emergency laryngostomy, and, my word, that would take some courage, then *heaven help you if your patient dies*.

So please, as well as learning the techniques thoroughly, just see how much cover your DHA will give you; a lot of you will be in for a shock... I know what my conscience would tell me to do, but it is easier to let your patient die isn't it?

FURTHER READING

Bradley, D. (1982) Minimum staffing levels on A & E units. *A & E News* (November).

Richardson, J.W. (Ed.) (1974) *Disaster planning*. Bristol: John Wright & Sons.

Savage, P.E.A. (1979) *Disasters. Hospital planning*, 1st edn. Oxford: Pergamon Press.

2 Reception and resuscitation of major emergencies

To get a full understanding of the principles involved in the care of the critically ill we must not start inside the accident and emergency department, but rather look from the scene of the incident, and then follow it through to the unit and it is to be hoped beyond. The ideal situation is that the critically ill patient is given immediate first aid by the ordinary man in the street. He is then taken swiftly by expertly trained and equipped ambulance men to a major accident unit and not, I must stress, not, to just any small hospital casualty. The accident and emergency department can only be as good as its specialist back-up. A small isolated hospital casualty department could probably give excellent care, but what then? There is no *fast* specialist back-up. Lives are wasted in many parts of the country every year because of this situation in which ambulances have to take critically injured patients to the nearest hospital rather than the most suitable. This is very old-fashioned thinking which is gradually, but all too slowly, changing in this country. Critically ill patients must bypass the smaller hospitals and be transported swiftly to major accident units with their full back-up facilities if more lives are to be saved.

The first hour after an injury must be thought of as a vital hour, a 'golden' hour. What happens in it will decide the patients very existence. Lethargy, indecision, too little treatment too late, will result in death. Prompt forceful resuscitation will give the patient every chance of life, and life of a better quality.

Let us look deeper now into the major link in the chain which concerns us in this book, that is, the accident and emergency department.

The emergency room

I consider that nothing in the whole field of nursing can match the challenge of the reception in the department of a major traumatic or medical emergency. None of your colleagues in any of their specialities have to have such wide ranging adaptability. For through those doors can come any conceivable emergency imaginable, at any time of the day or night. To cope efficiently with such a situation requires a very special type of person. Not everyone who wants to care for these patients will be able to cope with the stresses involved; you will only find out by trial and error if it suits you.

As a student or pupil you will at first be frightened about your ability to cope, this is quite natural and understandable and I would go as far as to say that if it does not occur you are foolhardy. By the end of your experience you should be able to cope fairly well with dire emergencies as long as trained nurses are working with you.

To be in charge of a resuscitation room for a span of duty is to have one of the most responsible jobs in the hospital because you must not only control yourself but your very words and movements must convey to those around you an air of calm so that they in turn will be able to give their best. This attitude, however, will only come to you with practical experience of countless emergencies. As a staff nurse or SEN on an accident and emergency unit you must then learn to cope on your own without a sister behind you suggesting what to do next. You must know what the doctor will want to do next and, in fact, have the confidence to tell the doctor what needs to be done next if he is very inexperienced.

Being prepared

The major principle of a resuscitation room is to *be prepared*. No matter how busy you are with existing emergencies, always have in the back of your mind that another might be on its way to you. Always have an emergency trolley free, always have resuscitation equipment available and ready for use, and always have it laid out tidily. It should be a perfect example of 'a place for everything and everything in its place'. By doing all these things, the chief enemy of the resuscitation room, *panic*, can be dealt a staggering blow.

Never trust any other person to have checked the emergency equipment. Check yourself at the start of each span of duty that every machine works, all connections are in the correct place, everything is within easy reach, brakes are on trolleys, oxygen cylinders are full, rubber is not perished, batteries are not dead, tubes/wires are not tangled, etc.

It is important in the general running of a resuscitation room that patients who do not require the facilities are placed in another part of the department. It is one of the trained nurse's main tasks to decide which patient to put where so that resuscitation is not blocked (triage).

A typical layout, with all the essential resuscitation equipment easily accessible for use without having to be moved, is shown in Fig. 5. Emergency equipment stored ready to be brought out is of little use; *it must be there on the spot and ready for use.* Another important point is that equipment must be easily visible. For

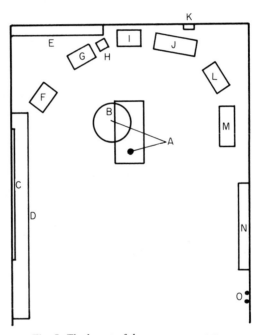

Fig. 5. *The layout of the emergency room.*

A	Accident trolley	I	Boyle's machine and respirator
B	Theatre light, and ceiling-mounted x-ray unit	J	Airway equipment and 'chest drain' kits
C	X-ray viewing boxes	K	Intercom, phones and stop-clock
D	Work surface	L	Intravenous infusion trolley
E	Stock of intravenous fluids	M	Dressings and suture materials
F	SWO and splint equipment	N	Emergency drugs
G	ECG monitor and defibrillator	O	Poles and scoop stretcher, plus a stool for external cardiac massage
H	Suction		

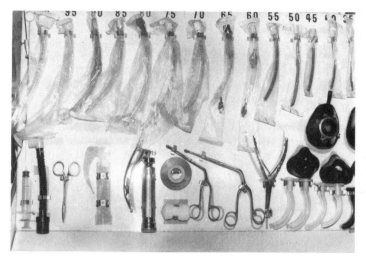

Fig. 6. *An excellent method of ensuring that emergency equipment is always available instantly.*

instance, having a laryngoscope hidden in some drawer or jumbled up with other items on a trolley is a time waster when time is essential. One way of overcoming this problem, which works very well is illustrated in Fig. 6. It is impossible to fail to notice missing equipment.

Certain drugs which are required immediately in an emergency (e.g. adrenaline, calcium chloride, sodium bicarbonate, isoprenaline, lignocaine and atropine) must be accessible. The location of the nearby key must be known by every member of the team.

One final point, someone, somewhere once stated 'If a piece of equipment is so made that it can be incorrectly used or fitted, sooner or later someone will do just that'. It's worth thinking about.

Delegation of tasks

A nurse leader must emerge who decides the priorities of treatment, delegates the tasks and then concentrates her efforts on the most demanding aspect at a particular time.

Initial assessment

As the patient comes through the door, look at the clothing for signs of damage that would indicate possible sites of injury. Look

at the position he is lying in. Talk to the ambulance crew and find
out these essentials:

1. What happened, in detail?
2. How was the patient when the ambulance arrived?
3. What injuries or conditions have they found already?
4. Do relations know that the patient is here?

A calm, controlled, confident and authoritative person should be
the only one to talk initially to the patient to reassure and let him

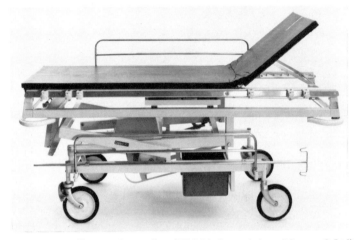

Fig. 7. *An excellent accident trolley.* (**With kind permission of Capecraft Ltd**)

know what is to happen. Avoid multiple questioning by a lot of
people.

Ask the patient what happened and where he is hurt. In a case
of trauma, go over the entire body before any clothes are
removed, asking about pain and seeing if the joints can move. This
gives you a complete picture of what has happened and the likely
injuries. Just to rush in removing clothes, albeit gently, is callous.

Place an identity bracelet on the patient at the earliest opportunity: this will prevent excessive questioning and help to prevent any
disastrous mix-up.

Lifting the patient

The patient should be lifted onto the accident trolley with either a scoop stretcher or poles and canvas (see Figs 189 and 190, p. 303). No seriously ill or injured patient should be 'man-handled' from one trolley to another unless orthopnoeic. If the patient is unconscious because of trauma or has any neck pain, carefully support the head and neck during transfer. A cervical collar may also be required. The accident unit trolley (Fig. 7) on which the patient is placed should have the following minimum specification:

1. Ability to tilt head down
2. Rigid x-ray translucent top
3. Efficient, attached, cot sides
4. Holders for intravenous infusions
5. Oxygen
6. Shelf for property
7. Back rest

The aim of a good accident and emergency service should be for the patient to be handled *once*, at the scene of the incident, onto a canvas or scoop and later, while still on that, lifted with poles or scoop onto an accident trolley. The patient should stay on that trolley right through the x-ray department and plaster room until arrival in the theatre or being placed on the bed. As little disturbance as possible helps, especially with a shocked or frightened patient.

Removal of clothing

Our first task is to remove clothing. This must be done completely so that the patient can be examined thoroughly. You will find that when injuries are overlooked it is because they are not searched for rather than simply missed in examination. I have seen a sock hide an ischaemic foot and a compound fracture and large wounds hidden under *intact* clothing. On many occasions patients will be certain that they do not have the slightest scratch on a particular limb; never take their word completely, always have a look.

A minimum of two nurses is required, more are ideal. Methods of removal vary and judgement comes only with experience. If speed is essential, large dressmaker's scissors complete the task

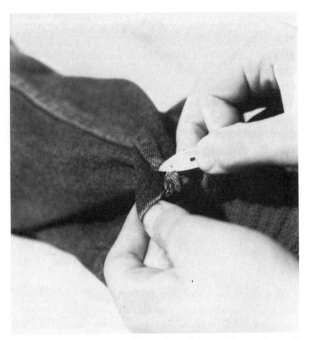

Fig. 8. *In an emergency clothes can be cut through in less than a minute. Generally, however, the seams may be cut through carefully using a scalpel.*

within a minute even through the thickest overcoat. But on most occasions excessive speed is quite unnecessary.

With more time on your hands the seams of clothes can be cut with a scalpel blade (Fig. 8). If major fractures are present the cut clothing can be left under the injured limb so that there is minimal disturbance to the patient.

When undressing the patient always take the good limb out of the clothing first, as you do with a hemiplegic patient on the wards. If buttons are undone first, all the upper clothes can often be removed easily by lifting both the patient's arms high above the head. Any first-aid wound dressing should be left on until the clothes have been removed. Ensure as much privacy for your patient as possible, but not at the expense of being able to see what you are doing or of gentleness. The utmost dexterity will be required for some of the elderly who have more layers of clothes than there are skins on an onion. The highest number of layers on a chest that I have seen is 13!

It may surprise you to know how many people would prefer to go through severe pain than to have their clothing damaged, so ask first. With a very resistant patient, pain can be eased with Entonox while removal continues.

Patients' property and valuables. This is a good point to mention patients' property and valuables. Suffice it to say that I can think of few occasions when patients have complained of the nursing care they have received; but there are many occasions when questions have arisen over property. The lesson to be learned, therefore, is that although the physical well-being of your patient must be first in your mind, you must make property and valuables a very close second and have witnesses to whatever you touch. Documentation will be required, depending on local policies.

The doctor's examination

If the patient has a medical condition a limited examination will be made by the doctor. However, if the patient has been injured, the whole of the body from head to toe will have to be examined. The examination will not be like those you see every day on the wards. In an accident and emergency unit there has to be a compromise between speed of examination, life-saving procedures and complete thoroughness, so that nothing is missed. We frequently have a situation in which treatment has to begin before a diagnosis is made. A doctor who spends half an hour examining a critically ill patient will one day have a dead patient, as will one who is too fast and misses injuries. Doctors inexperienced in casualty will need help and it is the nurse's duty to draw attention to anything that may be helpful. Look along with the doctor: two sets of critical eyes are better than one and by doing this you will soon become experienced in what to look out for.

Head. At the patient's head look and feel for lumps, bumps, lacerations and grazes among the hair. Notice any bleeding from the nose, ears and mouth. Look for facial asymmetry caused by either paralysis or swellings overlying fractures. Especially if there is a history of head injury, test pupil reactions and note the size.

Limbs. With the limbs compare both sides, notice the length, positions, bruises, swellings or grazes, all of which can point to a

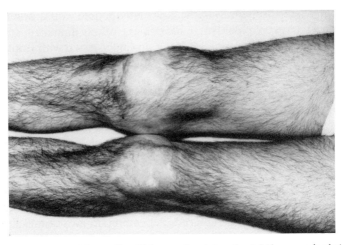

Fig. 9. *A fracture of the patella with haemarthrosis into the right knee, made obvious on comparison of the knees.*

bony injury. Fig. 9 shows the enlightening effect of comparison. The range of joint movements will also be tested.

Chest. When the chest is being examined look closely for paradoxical respiration. This is a flail area of chest wall overlying serious rib fractures, which moves in the opposite direction to the remaining chest. If noticed, mark the area with a pen so that it is not lost. Small localized areas of paradox will soon be hidden by swelling and may not be noticeable by the time the patient arrives on the ward. Look carefully for steering-wheel marks which can show up on the chest wall (Fig. 10). When lifting or rolling the patient over for the doctor, feel for the crackling of surgical emphysema. This is caused by air leaking from the lungs into the tissues of the chest wall. If very severe it can spread over the whole body making the patient look like a Michelin tyre man!

Abdomen. The abdomen, although soft, can still be bruised and grazed. This is especially noticeable in front-seat occupants of cars when in the impact of a crash, they have been forced against the seat belt, dashboard or steering-wheel. Look carefully for these marks and if found realize that enormous forces have acted to cause them and therefore suspect deep serious injuries. If serious abdominal injury is suspected, measure the abdomen with a tape measure and mark the level with a ball-point pen (Fig. 11); an increasing girth, although by no means conclusive, is an extra pointer to help the surgeon decide whether or not to do a laparotomy. Similarly, an increasing neck measurement can be a pointer towards haemorrhage from a ruptured arch of aorta.

Base-line

A base-line of the patient's condition has to be obtained as soon as possible after admission. This will include pulse, blood pressure, respirations, the level of consciousness and pupil reactions if there has been any head injury.

Next of kin

You must ask your patient about his next of kin and try to contact them. The police, friends or the patient's employers will often do

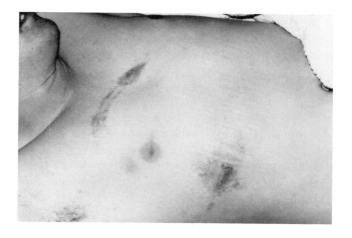

Fig. 10. *Marks made by a steering wheel on the patient's chest; he had multiple rib fractures.*

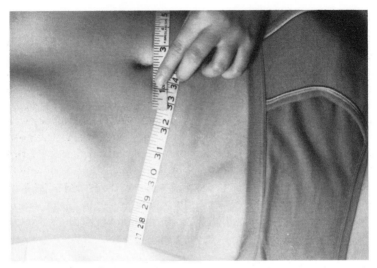

Fig. 11. *Measuring the abdominal girth; an increase in size is an extra pointer to the possibility of intra-abdominal haemorrhage.*

this for you but occasionally a telephone call is necessary. State briefly and reassuringly what has happened, and make sure they understand you and know where to come.

When relatives arrive, it is usually far more comforting for them to see the patient, despite the fact that they often get in the way, than just to be told about his condition. So first give the patient adequate preparation as regards tubes and drips and the like. As soon as the patient looks reasonable, go with the relatives to the bed-side while they say a brief 'hello'. Afterwards tea and a sit-down in a quiet room away from other people will help and frequently they will want to phone someone to ask them to come. Make it your business to go back to the room at intervals through the patient's stay in the department so that the relatives are kept up-to-date on the patient's progress, even if the news is bad. If the condition of a Roman Catholic patient is critical, bear in mind that a priest may have to be called; I have always found them to be of tremendous help and able to give comfort to relatives when my own words have been useless. Although not as frequently required, Church of England and non-conformist ministers can play a large part in giving both patients and relatives comfort and peace of mind.

Documentation

Documentation, although not a nurse's job, is something that you must bear in mind. It has to be done with speed and accuracy. Case papers ten minutes after the patient's admission are of no use. Papers are required within a few minutes so that the filling of blood bottles and the labelling of patients can be done safely. If, during a multiple accident, you are unsure of the identification of a patient, go to him and ask 'What is your name?' never 'Are you Mr ——?' An injured or sick person will occasionally not hear you and just say yes, trying to cooperate. I have known this to happen and the wrong patient has been sent to a ward. Make sure you know of this danger and that all your staff do as well.

Final check list

With major emergencies so many things require doing all at the same time that the routine items are often forgotten until after the patient has left the department (Fig. 12). Have a mental check list of items such as:

Does your patient have any drug allergies?
Is the patient covered for tetanus?
Have all the listed treatments been carried out, wounds cleaned and injections given?
Are the ward staff ready for the patient?
Do the laboratory know which ward the patient is going to?
Have the clerks completed all the final documentation?
Are radiographs going with the patient?
Any ECGs?
Have relatives been informed?
Is all property safe, including false teeth?

RESUSCITATION

This section is intended not only for nurses working in a major accident unit surrounded by doctors but also for those working in isolation, perhaps in a peripheral hospital where it may be five to ten minutes before the doctor arrives. It is essential that specialist accident and emergency nurses realize the 'fill-in' role they must often play and are fully conversant with advanced resuscitation techniques. Patients' very lives depend on it.

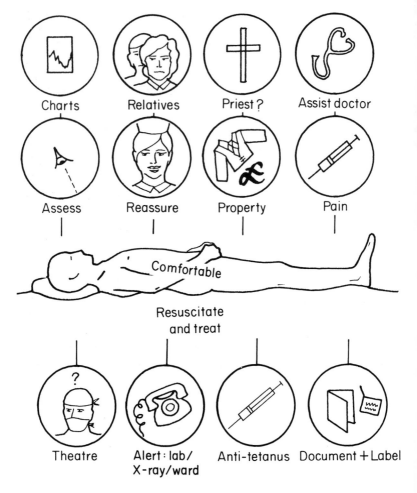

Charts **Relatives** **Priest?** **Assist doctor**

Assess **Reassure** **Property** **Pain**

Comfortable

Resuscitate
and treat

Theatre **Alert: lab/ X-ray/ward** **Anti-tetanus** **Document + Label**

Fig. 12. *Nursing routines for the reception of major trauma.*

The initial assessment

As the patient is wheeled in, an instantaneous assessment of the patient's condition is made and you ask yourself four questions (Fig. 13):

1. Does the patient have a carotid pulse?
2. Is the patient breathing?

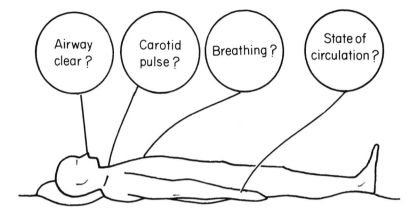

Fig. 13. *The initial assessment of the patient.*

3. If the patient is breathing, is the airway clear?
4. Does the patient have a satisfactory circulation?

Nurses are used to feeling for a pulse at the wrist and seldom miss; practice is therefore required so that the carotid pulse can be located, first time, every time, in an emergency situation (Fig. 14).

While you feel for the pulse, watch the chest for respiratory movement, listen for the sound of breathing and feel for breath from the mouth. Also, simultaneously, you must look at the skin colour, see the state of the veins, whether collapsed or full, and decide if the patient is shocked.

I must stress that *you must find the answer to these four questions within seconds of the patient's arrival* and act decisively on what you find.

In an emergency there are two major catastrophes that you often meet:

1. Cardiac arrest
2. The unconscious patient with an obstructed airway

Let us look at how you, as a nurse, must deal with them. Once you have mastered the techniques in this section and are able to adapt them to other situations, then you will be surprised how self-confident you will be and how much better able to cope with the many forms of trauma which at any moment could come through the admission door.

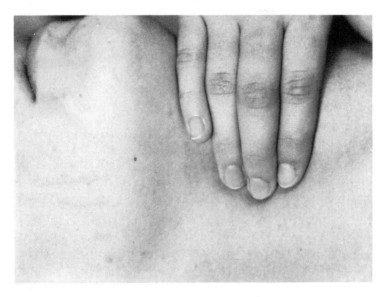

Fig. 14. *Finding the carotid pulse.*

CARDIAC ARREST

Perhaps *the* ultimate emergency is cardiac arrest. Literally every second counts. Although it would be impossible to plot a truly accurate graph of your patient's chances of survival, the graph in Fig. 15 gives a fair idea of how quickly you must act.

External cardiac massage is the first essential, the ambulance must be met at the door and the attendants assisted while the patient is taken by trolley into the department. While the patient is being lifted onto the accident trolley, the department team takes over the resuscitation, each setting about her predetermined job as follows:

Removing essential clothing
External cardiac massage (ECM)
Ventilating the lungs
Getting an intravenous line into the patient
Obtaining a monitor trace
Preparing drugs

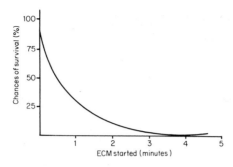

Fig. 15. *A graph showing how essential it is for survival to start resuscitation as soon as possible.*

The ambulance attendants must not leave at this stage; their presence is essential both to help to provide information such as how the incident occurred, how the patient was when they arrived at the scene, what they have done, what response there has been, whether there are any relatives or friends and the like. Greater involvement of ambulance personnel in this type of situation is a major factor in their ability to resuscitate patients more effectively in the future.

Let us now go through the preceding list of procedures in detail.

Technique of external cardiac massage (ECM)

The first procedure to perform is external cardiac massage; even if the patient has stopped breathing some oxygen remains in the blood stream and this will be available for the tissues to use if only it can be pumped round the body. The design of the heart's valvular system is such that simple compression will pump blood round the body. In external cardiac massage we press directly over the lower end of the sternum using the heel of one hand placed directly over the other (Fig. 16). The degree of compression of the chest is about 4 cm (Fig. 17), achieved by a backwards and forwards rocking motion, the elbows being kept extended. This action must be continued rhythmically about 60 times a minute. It is extremely tiring and helpers will be necessary if it is kept up for any length of time. Everyone, short or tall, will find a footstool a great help, or, if possible, you may kneel on the trolley. Some machines are available to perform external cardiac massage for you!

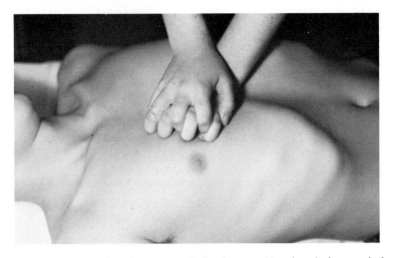

Fig. 16. *For external cardiac massage the hands are positioned on the lower end of the sternum.*

Ventilating the lungs

Before the lungs can be inflated the airway has to be cleared; this is dealt with in detail later in the chapter.

Inflating the lungs can be done in several ways but the insertion of a cuffed endotracheal tube is the method of choice; this (*a*) ensures a clear airway and (*b*) will protect the lungs from gastric contents. Nearly all cases of cardiac arrest occurring outside the hospital have vomit in the pharynx. In well over 50 per cent of

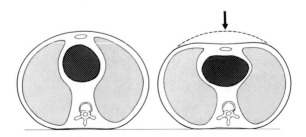

Fig. 17. *The pressure during external cardiac massage compresses the chest about 4 cm and thus squeezes the heart between the sternum and the vertebrae.*

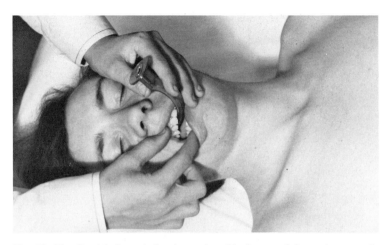

Fig. 18. *The Guedel airway is first inserted upside down and then, when near the back of the mouth, inverted.*

these cases ECM has caused considerable gastric emptying making intubation of paramount importance. However, it is often best for the inexperienced nurse in the first instance to insert a Guedel airway (Fig. 18) and 'bag' the patient with air or oxygen. This is done alternately with external cardiac massage in a ratio of about six chest compressions to one lung inflation. Bagging the patient in this way, even when using a comparatively simple device such as the Ambu, is no easy feat. It is important to get an air-tight seal around the nose and mouth, keep the head extended and pull the jaw forward, all at the same time (Fig. 19). Another complication with the Ambu or similar bag is that the high pharyngeal pressures involved will mean that a fair amount of air is forced down the oesophagus, distending the patients stomach. This can lead to expulsion of stomach contents during ECM.

Intubation is essentially a practical skill which should be taught first in the classroom and on models, then on patients under the strictest supervision. The technique should be well within the capabilities of the specialist accident and emergency nurse (further notes on the technique are supplied in Appendix I).

The operator will usually require the patient to be flat on his back with a pillow under the head. A full range of endotracheal tubes must be available. However, as a very rough guide, a size 9.5 mm will be reasonable for most fully grown men and a size 8.5 mm

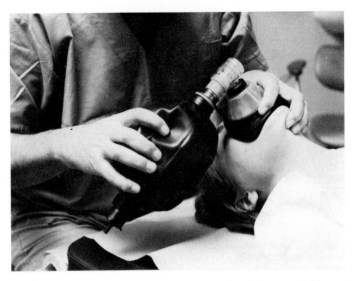

Fig. 19. *Holding the face-mask with the head extended and the jaw pulled forward to keep the airway clear.* (**With kind permission of Ambu International**)

for women. Test the cuff on the tube by inflating it with air before it is handed to the operator. The exclusive use of disposable tubes in emergency work will cut down the chances of a tube with a faulty cuff being used.

Another technique which is little used on this side of the Atlantic is the insertion of the oesophageal obturator airway (Fig. 20). This is inserted 'blind' like a stomach tube well down into the oesophagus. A balloon at the end is then inflated inside the oesophagus to prevent regurgitation of stomach contents into the airway. Air or oxygen can then be introduced via the tube into the pharynx and then into the trachea. Unlike endotracheal tubes, it can be used after very little practice and would certainly seem to have a future place in our accident and emergency departments for use by trained nurses while they acquire proficiency in endo-tracheal intubation.

Suction may be required by the operator at any moment and the equipment should therefore be ready to be placed in his hand. During the procedure pressure over the cricoid cartilage in the neck may be required (Fig. 21). Once the tube has been intro-

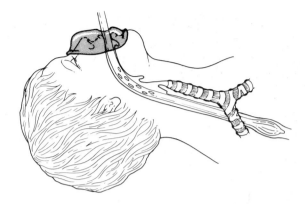

Fig. 20. *The oesophageal obturator airway.*

duced, secure it in position with tape or bandage (Fig. 22) and ensure that the connecting tube does not drag on the endotracheal tube. The three absolute essentials have now been accomplished, that is, by now you have or should have:

A major pulse that is palpable
The lungs being inflated
A clear airway

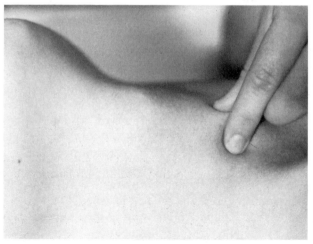

Fig. 21. *Exerting pressure over the cricoid cartilage.*

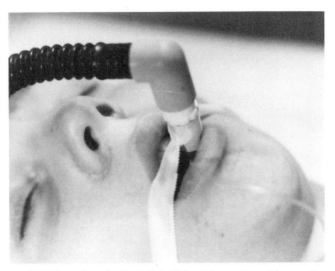

Fig. 22. *The endotracheal tube is held firmly in position with strapping.*

Recent work in the USA has suggested that increased intrathoracic pressure caused by ECM and ventilation being performed simultaneously has resulted in an increased cardiac output, so you may see continuous ECM and ventilation being tried more frequently in the future.

Intravenous infusion

The next task, which may be done simultaneously depending on staff availability, is to get an intravenous infusion running (the 'motorway' into the body for drugs). No time is wasted undressing the patient or getting his arm out of a coat. You must simply cut through the sleeves. Even in a patient with cardiac arrest, as long as external cardiac massage is being performed correctly, a vein should easily be brought up with a tourniquet on a dependent limb within a few seconds. Sodium bicarbonate 8.4% is the fluid of choice, 50 ml being run in at the first instance, followed by 30 ml over the next five minutes. The vein is then kept open by 5% dextrose. Venepuncture, like intubation, is not universally accepted as a nursing procedure. The skill is, however, of primary importance to the accident and emergency nurse *in the emergency situation*. It must be learned and practised, so that it can be done with efficiency and speed when the need arises. The antecubital fossa, the radial border of the forearm and the dorsum of the hand are the sites with which nurses are most familiar and are therefore the best sites for them to use (further details of the techniques are supplied in Appendix II).

Monitoring the patient

Obtaining a monitor reading is the next consideration. Many different makes of monitor are available, but a very quick reading can be obtained directly from the defibrillator paddles of a Life Aid. Alternatively, the normal four-limb electrodes can be attached or electrodes can be stuck on to the chest.

When connected, the monitor should show one of the following tracings (Fig. 23):

1. Ventricular fibrillation
2. Asystole
3. Ventricular stand-still
4. Normal ECG

If coarse ventricular fibrillation is present, *defibrillation* will be the next step. Defibrillation, however, will be of no use if asystole shows on the monitor. Some authorities believe, quite reasonably, that it is best to defibrillate at the outset in all cases of arrest because most arrests are in ventricular fibrillation and the longer defibrillation is left the less likely it is to be successful. The chest is first greased with electrode jelly or, preferably, two electrically conductive pads can be placed over the areas to prevent your hand slipping while you do external cardiac message. The position of the paddles is shown in Fig. 24.

If you are the 'nurse leader' present, make doubly sure that no one is in contact with the patient, trolley or equipment while the shock is being given and that the patient is not touching any metallic part of the trolley.

About *100 to 200 joules* are given for the initial shock and, if that is not successful, the shock will probably be repeated at a higher level, up to 400 joules. However, recent US research suggests that large shocks of up to 400 joules are inappropriate.

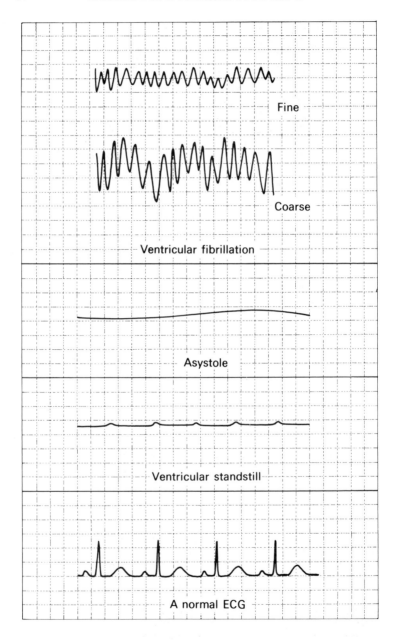

Fig. 23. *Ventricular fibrillation, asystole, ventricular standstill and normal ECG.*

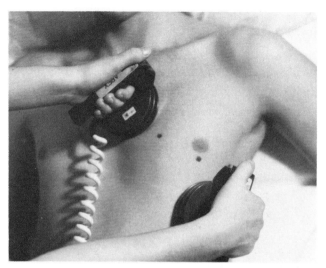

Fig. 24. *The position of the defibrillator paddles.*

Drugs

The final consideration in cardiac arrest is drugs. These will vary enormously with the patient's condition and the doctors concerned, but the list shown in Table 1 should meet the needs of most and serve as a general guide to the drugs which should be

Table 1. *Some drugs used during and after a cardiac arrest.*

Adrenaline 1 : 1000	Verapamil hydrochloride 5 mg
Calcium chloride 10%	Bretylium tosylate 100 mg
Calcium gluconate 10%	Salbutamol 5 mg
Atropine 600 μg	Heparin
Isoprenaline 2 mg	Diamorphine hydrochloride (heroin) 5 mg
Lignocaine 2% and 20%	Pethidine 100 mg
Sodium bicarbonate 8.4%	Potassium chloride 20%
Hydrocortisone 100 mg	Practolol 10 mg
Frusemide 20 mg and 250 mg	Dopamine hydrochloride 200 mg
Digoxin 500 μg	Propranolol 1 mg
Ouabain 0.25 mg	Prochlorperazine 12.5 mg
Aminophylline 250 mg	Dextrose 5% 500 ml
Diazepam 10 mg	Disopyramide 100 mg

available for the general resuscitation of any patient. Of all the drugs listed, the three in use for most cases of arrest are:

A drip of 8.4% sodium bicarbonate
Adrenaline 1 : 1000
Calcium chloride 10%

These are well worth while preparing if an arrested patient is expected.

Appendix III mentions the actions of some of the drugs listed, and Fig. 25 recaps on the main points of cardiac arrest procedure.

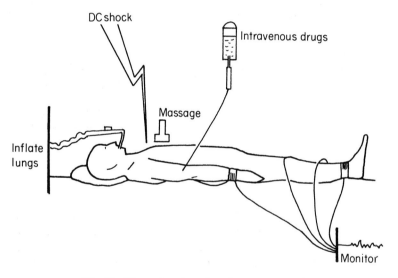

Fig. 25. *The main points of cardiac arrest procedure.*

UNCONSCIOUS PATIENT WITH AN OBSTRUCTED AIRWAY

The other major critical emergency is the unconscious patient with an obstructed airway. Once again it is something with which you must learn to cope on your own, perhaps for many minutes until further help arrives. Throughout your time in the accident and emergency department you are bound to see many such patients. The routine of what must be done to aid them includes:

- Position the patient on his side with the head low
- Clean out the mouth and pharynx and *sometimes* remove the false teeth
- Insert an airway and pull jaw forwards
- Extend the head minimally and with extreme care if there is the possibility of a cervical spine injury

Let us now deal with each of these points individually.

The patient is first of all positioned on his side (Fig. 26); this position and its variations have had many names over the years (recovery, lateral, coma, tonsillectomy, three-quarter prone and unconscious) but I think saying 'get the patient on his side' carries the message clearly enough. Being on his side will assist any blood,

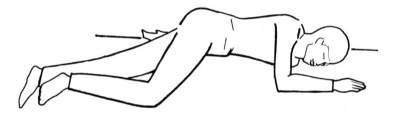

Fig. 26. *The coma position.*

vomitus, saliva or the like to trickle out of the mouth rather than to run into the pharynx and block the airway. Lowering the head end of the trolley is the next thing to do since this enhances the 'downhill run' to the lips for any fluid in the mouth. If your patient is drunk and unconscious, with a head injury, and vomiting literally pints of beer, no suction machine in the world will be able to cope and simply putting the patient over in this position is life-saving.

The mouth is then opened and the whole of the mouth and pharynx cleaned out by suction or wiping.

If the patient has false teeth which are easily removed, it is best if they are taken out. Remember that small plates which can easily fall to the back of the mouth are far more dangerous than full sets. If the situation arises, and it often will, where the jaws are firmly clenched together, it may prove easier, for you and the patient, if the teeth are left in. *Never stick doggedly to a rule without thinking carefully and weighing up the 'pros and cons'; all patients are different.*

Even with jaws clenched together the mouth can be sucked out between the teeth and the pharynx by use of a soft suction catheter via the nose. If breathing becomes worse it is also worth a trial of a nasal airway. In all unconscious patients the insertion of a Ryle's tube will help to prevent the airway being further endangered.

If access to the mouth becomes urgent, a Ferguson mouth gag (Fig. 27) can be used, although this can be very traumatic. Alternatively, if time permits, two wooden spatulas can be inserted more gently and others inserted one at a time between these two to widen the gap between the teeth (Fig. 28). This latter method is useful where the patient's tongue is firmly trapped between the teeth and you can safely afford to spend a minute or two to free it slowly and gently.

At this stage, I would like to mention that I would like to see nurses make more use of the laryngoscope, a very under-used instrument, thought of by most purely as a tool for intubation. Nothing could be further from the truth, since it is invaluable for visualization while sucking out the pharynx. For most accident and emergency work a rigid Yankauer type of suction catheter is best because it gives positive control of position and does not collapse.

The third item on our initial list is insertion of an airway and pulling the jaw forwards. The Guedel airway is usually inserted upside down at first until the tip touches the top of the hard palate (see Fig. 18). It is then twisted through 180° and inserted until in place. Suction can then be carried out through the airway with a soft catheter. Kink the suction tube while it is being introduced and only suck while it is being withdrawn. Do this in short bursts rather than in prolonged sessions, so that the patient can be adequately oxygenated in between times. On some occasions the patient's level of unconsciousness will be so light that he will still have a 'gag' reflex and an airway will cause more harm than good, making the patient retch and vomit. If this is case, leave just the end of the airway between the teeth or part of the way down. With an unconscious patient who has a head injury, beware of the head hanging too low and causing 'kinking' of the neck veins. This can increase intracranial bleeding and worsen cerebral oedema; to avoid it place a small pillow under the head. Lifting the jaw

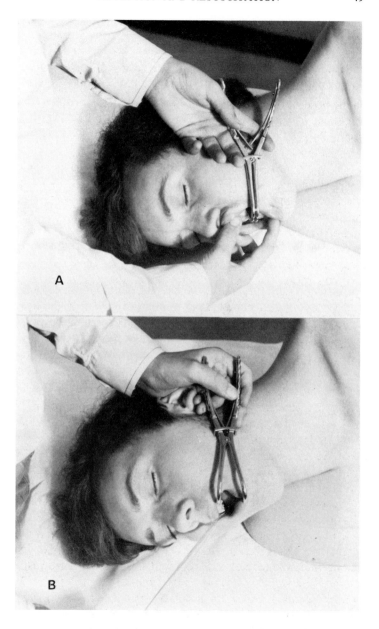

Fig. 27. *The use of the Ferguson mouth gag.* **A**, insertion; **B**, opened.

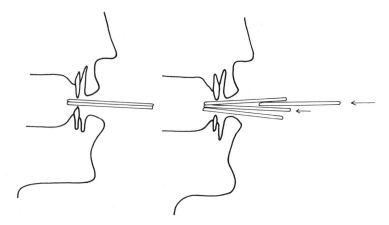

Fig. 28. *Using a series of wooden spatulas to open clenched jaws.*

forwards lifts the tongue off the back of the pharynx, helping the airway even more. Finally, bear in mind extension of the head as being very useful if there is no obvious cervical spine injury; this lifts the tongue farther off the back of the pharynx (Fig. 29) and can make all the difference between quiet and obstructed breathing.

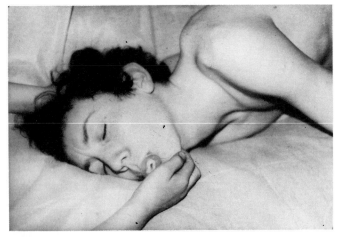

Fig. 29. *Extending the head and pulling the jaw forward to clear the airway.*

Never leave your unconscious patients alone, even for a moment. Inhalation of vomit can occur very quietly and unless you are alert it will be missed, until the patient turns blue!

If your patient has had a period of anoxia, oxygen can now be given until he is pink again, but remember that it is of secondary importance. An obstructed airway needs clearing first.

Intubation of the unconscious patient is a completely different problem from the procedure in an arrested patient. With an arrest you have a flaccid, lifeless patient; here you have a far more difficult situation, with the patient often rolling about, grinding teeth and clenching jaws. Although intubation is often very important and beneficial, it can usually be delayed until a skilled anaesthetist arrives by using the methods just mentioned. I have on two occasions had to intubate while waiting for a doctor, but in these cases they were literally failing in front of my eyes and there was no time to wait.

CHOKING

In an accident and emergency situation we tend to see the end result of choking, i.e. cardio/respiratory arrest, rather than a

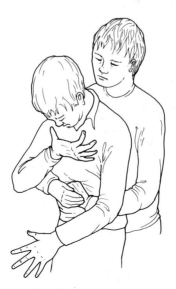

Fig. 30. *The Heimlich manoeuvre.*

patient clutching his throat and going blue. However, just in case you do come across a patient in whom it is just occurring, I would like to mention an effective procedure called the Heimlich manoeuvre which is easy to carry out. You stand behind the patient (Fig. 30) clasping your hands together so that the fist of one is pointing towards the patient's abdomen; then give a sharp thrust, something like a bear hug. This has the effect of increasing the intrathoracic pressure because the abdominal organs press against the diaphragm.

Variations of this technique are possible while the patient is lying face upwards or on his side and can also be tried, together with the long established back slapping.

If these comparatively simple methods fail, the doctor will have to use the laryngoscope and Magill forceps as the patient lapses into unconsciousness.

FURTHER READING

Harber, T. & Lucas, B.G.B. (1980) An evaluation of some mechanical resuscitators. *Annals of the Royal College of Surgeons of England*, 62.

3 Care of major traumatic emergencies

The study of injuries of the head, chest and abdomen can be intensely interesting, yet death can follow far more swiftly than with any orthopaedic trauma. Non-orthopaedic emergencies are, however, a sadly neglected section of accident care. Look along the bookshelves of a medical library and you will understand what I mean. The traumatologist has to be experienced, decisive and act promptly if life is to be saved. You must be acutely observant and match his skills. With an exsanguinated patient, your actions in the emergency room during the first half an hour or so will decide whether the patient lives or dies.

First of all let me mention a few points about bleeding which many nurses just do not realize.

1. Bleeding does not usually occur *all at once*; it is often a progressive process which can continue for hours or days.
2. A patient with internal bleeding is in far more danger than one with a surface wound or an amputation, because the urgency of the situation is not realized as easily.
3. A patient can lose blood and, for a while, still maintain a reasonable pulse and blood pressure because of the body's defence mechanisms.

Add together these features and you have a potentially fatal situation, where a patient can be losing blood rapidly internally, have a reasonable pulse and blood pressure and look just a little pale.

Base-line

As soon as possible after admission a pulse and blood pressure 'base-line' must be obtained on which to judge later readings. However, a central venous pressure line will give a far more accurate estimate of the patient's blood volume even before the pulse and blood pressure show any change. As a general rule blood loss tends to be underestimated. Blood must be taken for grouping and cross-matching. If there are multiple casualties be 101 per cent sure of the details on the blood bottles; in an emergency mistakes are far more likely to occur and it is every-one's responsibility to ensure that none are made.

Central venous pressure line (CVP)

Even in the few years since the first edition of this book the CVP line has changed from being used only occasionally in our depart-ments, to being a commonly used diagnostic procedure.

Under strict aseptic conditions a catheter is placed in a large neck vein and passed until it is positioned in the large veins at the entrance to the right atrium of the heart. We can thus get a very accurate measure of the pressure in these veins and therefore of the amount of blood which the patient has in his circulation. Normal values are from 5 to 10 mm H_2O. In shock it will be less than 5 mm H_2O.

The CVP is only measured intermittently. In the intervening periods the CVP catheter is left connected to an ordinary line for giving blood or fluids. Because of the catheter's large bore it is ideal for giving rapid transfusions.

Intravenous infusion

Bear in mind that it is far easier to take down an unnecessary infusion or take out a cannula than it is to put one up in the x-ray department on a severely shocked patient with collapsed veins. Most casualties, when first admitted, have veins which can be 'brought up' within a minute with a tourniquet and intravenous cut-downs are rarely necessary; this will not hold true by the time the patient has been 'processed'. The lesson, therefore, is to get an infusion or i.v. cannula such as a Venflon under way sooner rather than later, and to think what blood loss the patient might have soon if some of the aches and pains turn out to be due to fractures or ruptured organs.

An intravenous infusion will in all probability be one of the earliest treatments, if not the first, to be given to a seriously injured patient. As mentioned earlier, it is best done on admission *before* the veins collapse. Finding a vein for the doctor is an art in itself. Many failures are due to impatience and ignorance of simple techniques. Place a tourniquet round the patient's arm and have the arm hanging down over the side of the trolley; get a good light on the site and briskly stroke the arm upwards. If the patient can help, ask him to open and close the hand as this will encourage blood flow. Finally, flicking over the proposed injection site will help to make the veins stand out. Do not give up if nothing appears immediately, be patient. Leave the tourniquet on and look again in about a minute. If nothing shows suggest a large neck vein. A cut-down is very rarely necessary. With massive blood loss several sites will be required, both above and below the diaphragm, to get in the enormous amounts of blood and fluid required.

Once the infusion is up, do not allow all the work to be in vain; secure it well. If it is on a joint splint it well. Never underestimate the strength of an unconscious patient's arm; the drip can be out in seconds. If the patient is restless, ask someone to hold the arm and do nothing else; another vein may be hard to find. For further details see Appendix II.

Control of surface haemorrhage

Very severe surface haemorrhage obviously occurs, but let us not overplay its part. It is quite a rarity, seldom occurring even once a month in an average department. Control is achieved in 99 per cent of cases by direct pressure and elevation of the part.

Let us now go into this aspect in a little more detail. Firstly, your patient should be lying down and you should talk and reassure him constantly, remembering that the best reassurance you can give is to demonstrate by the firmness of your actions that he is in good hands. Open pads and mosquito forceps onto a dressing pack in readiness. Even in the most atrocious wounds you will find that the bulk of the bleeding is from one or perhaps two major points. Bearing this in mind, peel off the sodden first-aid dressing slowly and be guided by any history which the ambulance men have given you. If there is a history of arterial haemorrhage in a limb, put a pneumatic tourniquet round the limb so that it is ready to inflate if necessary. Once the bleeding is met, find exactly where it is coming from and press with your finger directly over the gauze on the site for several minutes. The doctor will then be able to examine the wound as you lift the dressing off. After the doctor has seen it, cover once again and bandage firmly in position. If haemorrhage re-starts while the wound is uncovered, or has never stopped, first try direct local pressure (Fig. 31) to part of the wound so that the doctor can examine it well and ensure that no nerves or vessels are damaged. If the doctor still cannot see the wound properly, apply the tourniquet for a few moments. When it has been looked at, redress and rebandage it well, then release the tourniquet. It is almost unknown for direct pressure not to stop the haemorrhage *if correctly applied over the bleeding site*.

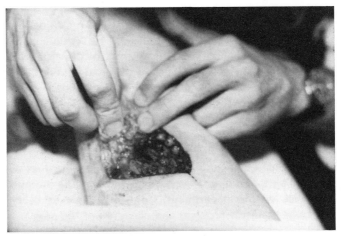

Fig. 31. *Direct local pressure to the wound will stop haemorrhages in 99 per cent of cases.*

THE SHOCKED PATIENT

The word 'shock', despite much teaching, is still both over-used and misused. I do, however, prefer to use it because of its simplicity. Shock is basically inadequate perfusion of the tissues of the vital organs. It is usually associated with general physical collapse of the patient. In trauma the main causes are loss of whole blood or plasma.

Recognition is essential. I have seen many patients die of haemorrhage, but in very few of those instances have I been able to *see* the blood which was lost. This is because it was internal haemorrhage and something which if you cannot see you are not always aware of. Let me give you an example of this. Look at Fig. 32. Felt has been wrapped round the person's body to represent a blood loss of about 50 per cent or more. See how it blends in with the body contours and is difficult to see. See also how it is easily covered up by clothing, making assessment at the site of an accident even more difficult. Blood loss which you cannot see is therefore a dangerous situation (Fig. 33).

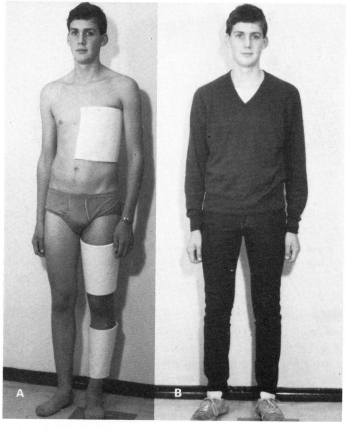

Fig. 32. A, *Felt attached to the body representing a blood loss of about 50 per cent. Notice that it hardly affects the body contours.* **B**, *beneath clothes the loss is invisible.*

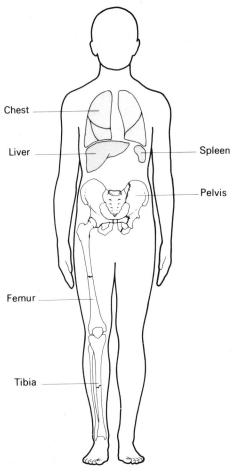

Fig. 33. *Common sites of 'hidden' blood loss.*

People can bleed to death in front of you without a drop of blood being seen. The least obvious injuries are frequently the most life threatening. Radiographs are partly to blame for nurses not realizing fully the implications of internal haemorrhage. Radiographs show you bones and it is easy to forget the huge mass of vascular tissue which surrounds them. After a fracture, the bone ends, if displaced, rip through the muscles producing blood loss, and hence you see the progressive swelling round fractures (Fig. 34). Assuming that we cannot see the blood loss, the list below tells you how to recognize a shocked patient:

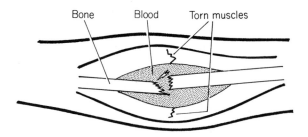

Bone   Blood   Torn muscles

Fig. 34. *Bleeding from the fracture site is a common cause of shock.*

1. A large element of suspicion and experience is involved in knowing that a particular patient may well become shocked soon because of the injuries or history of the accident.
2. The pulse will become progressively more rapid and feeble.
3. The skin will become pale, cold and clammy, and the surface veins on the body will be collapsed and difficult to see.
4. The blood pressure will eventually fall, although a far earlier warning is given by the central venous pressure (CVP).
5. There may be air hunger.
6. The patient may become increasingly restless and drowsy.

The condition should be recognized and the doctor called by the time that item 3 is realized.

Treatment is, of course, by transfusion of whole blood as soon as this becomes available. In the meantime, as a 'fill-in', HPPF, Dextran or Haemaccel can be used. In exsanguinated patients be prepared for the transfusions to be rapid and frequent, for instance 500 ml in about five minutes. Thirty two units of fluid in one hour is the maximum which I personally have seen. Use of the Travenol pump is ideal (Fig. 35). In a situation where many units of blood are being given rapidly, blood-warmers (Fig. 36) will be necessary to avert the danger of the heart arresting. This can be clamped to the drip stands and can accompany the patient to theatre or a ward.

Medical anti-shock trousers (MAST)

Another technique for treating shock, which is much favoured in America but is slow to catch on in this country, is the use of MAST (Fig. 37). These are placed under the patient, wrapped round his

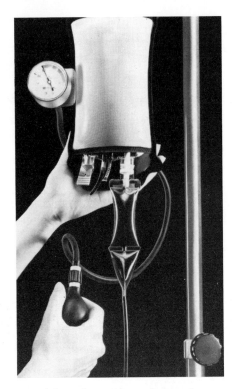

Fig. 35. *The pressure infuser for rapid transfusion when no spare hands are available.* (**With kind permission of Travenol Laboratories**)

lower legs and abdomen (looking like a pair of trousers) and firmly fastened. They are then inflated with compressed air to squeeze blood from the large veins in the legs and pelvis, into the upper part of the body and so to the vital organs.

Such a procedure will have the equivalent effect of a blood transfusion of up to 30 per cent of the body's circulating volume. There is also the added advantage that the pressure itself helps to close down the bleeding vessels.

The MAST are applied by the ambulance crew 'at the roadside' and left inflated. On arrival at the accident and emergency department the major problem with them is the danger of an inexperienced doctor or nurse taking them off before the patient has had some volume replacement. This is because as soon as they are removed the blood pressure can fall dramatically leaving an exsanguinated patient with impossible veins.

In some cases the MAST may have to stay on the patient until he goes into theatre and the surgeon is ready to make an incision.

The ideal method of removal is to slowly release the pressure over a period of half an hour to an hour as the blood volume is being replaced.

The other main considerations for large transfusions are as follows:

• O Rh-negative blood (the so called universal donor) will be needed in very urgent cases where there is simply no time for group and cross-match. This, however, is a life-saving only procedure.

• Special micro-filters will be required to remove microscopic

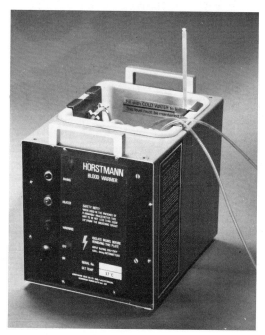

Fig. 36. *The Bristol blood-warmer, Mark II.* (**With kind permission of the Horstmann Gear Group**)

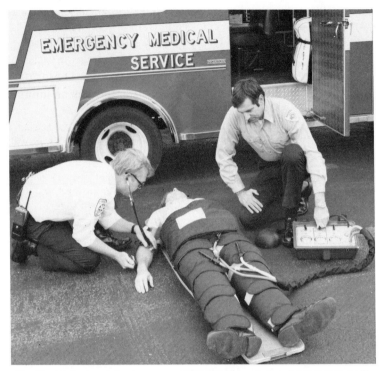

Fig. 37. *Medical anti-shock trousers.* (**With kind permission of J.O.B.S.T. Ltd**)

'sludge' from the the stored blood which would otherwise cause micro-emboli in the lungs and then respiratory distress.

- Platelets and other clotting factors quickly become useless in stored blood and this, added to the dilution which will occur as transfusion progresses, means that the factors will need to be replaced with fresh frozen plasma.
- Calcium gluconate may be required to combat citrate toxicity, and sodium bicarbonate needed for some acidosis.

ABDOMINAL INJURIES

If you have a shocked patient in front of you after an accident, and the amount of blood lost is estimated to exceed by far what could come from the injuries that have already been found, there must be blood in the chest or abdomen.

Look for the commonest injuries first. Damage to the spleen is the most common cause of blood loss, followed by damage to the liver. Both of these injuries are occasionally accompanied by a fracture or bruising over the lower ribs. The spleen can be particularly troublesome, only pouring out the blood hours or even days later. Tell the doctor of every instance when an injured patient complains of abdominal pain or discomfort, even if it is only momentary. Remember also that the pain can be referred to the shoulder and will require correct interpretation. Measurement of the girth (as mentioned in Chapter 2) is worth while, especially if the patient is unconscious.

Peritoneal lavage is now well accepted as the major way of deciding if a patient has an intra-abdominal haemorrhage.

The patient's bladder is emptied. Then under local anaesthetic the skin in the midline below the umbilicus is incised to the peritoneum and the trocar and cannula are inserted. The trocar is then removed and the drip set loaded with a litre of normal saline is connected up and run into the abdominal cavity. After a few minutes the fluid is syphoned out again by placing the drip bag on the bottom of the trolley. If the returned fluid is bloodstained a laparotomy will be required.

Other abdominal injuries seen fairly frequently include:

1. Retroperitoneal haematoma
2. Tears of the intestines and mesentery
3. Tears of major veins
4. Ruptured diaphragm

CHEST INJURIES

Since my wife has asthma, I can testify how frightening it is for patients not to be able to get their breath. No matter what else is wrong, severe breathlessness will be foremost in their minds. Several things can be done to ease a patient's plight. If conscious, most patients will prefer to sit up on the trolley and often to lean forward with arms raised on the cot sides. Many also hold the side of the chest which is affected.

A flail segment (Fig. 38), which occurs with double fractures of some ribs or isolated fractures of many ribs, is first treated by pressing firmly on the segment which moves paradoxically, there-

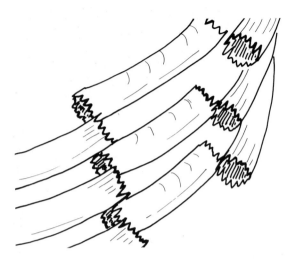

Fig. 38. *A flail segment in the chest wall.*

by stopping it from flopping about as the patient breathes. This, however, is a temporary measure and if the area is large, intubation and intermittent positive pressure ventilation (IPPV) will shortly be necessary. This will be followed at a later date by tracheostomy.

A pneumothorax is one of the commonest of all the serious chest injuries. Small ones can be left to absorb themselves and the lung to re-expand, but with one of any appreciable size a chest drain will be necessary (Fig. 39). The drain is best inserted in the second intercostal space in the mid-clavicular line. If blood is present (haemothorax) a drain is inserted low down at the sixth intercostal space at the mid-axillary line. A tension pneumothorax is an extreme emergency, the heart and great vessels being pushed over towards the opposite side preventing the 'good' lung from operating effectively. This patient, instead of having moderate distress as in an ordinary pneumothorax, will be extremely dyspnoeic and cyanosed as the condition progresses. He will deteriorate rapidly and die unless the air is released with great speed. With both of the previously mentioned drains a Heimlich flutter valve will be necessary to prevent back-flow of fluid and air into the pleural space (Fig. 40). The end of the tube leads to a drainage

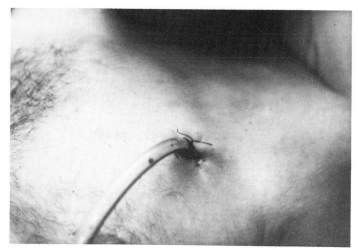

Fig. 39. *The tubing of an underwater seal drain connected to the left side of the chest.*

bag which has a measuring scale. Underwater seal bottles are not really ideal for an accident and emergency unit where the patient is being moved from time to time. Quite frankly, there are just too many things which can go wrong with them. However, they remain in common use.

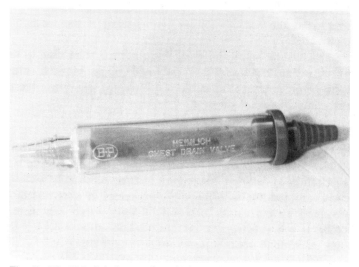

Fig. 40. *The Heimlich flutter valve which may be attached to the chest drain.*

Patients with severe pain from multiple rib fractures can conveniently be given oxygen and analgesia at the same time using Entonox. This contains 50% oxygen, which is about 30 per cent more than is in ordinary air and is therefore beneficial.

Immediate emergency tracheostomy has no part to play in the accident and emergency department, except perhaps for:

1. Oedema round the larynx
2. A foreign body which cannot be removed

Chest wounds

Penetrating wounds of the chest wall can sometimes allow air to be sucked in and blown out with each respiration (sucking wound). Temporary treatment of this is to seal off the wound with an air-tight dressing and possibly insertion of a temporary underwater seal chest drain into the chest via the wound. Thoracotomy will then be necessary as soon as is feasible.

Cardiac tamponade is usually the result of a knife wound. Following injury blood collects under the pericardium, pressing in on the heart and therefore preventing it from filling and pumping as it should. You therefore have a patient with a rapid, weak pulse and raised or normal central venous pressure. Pericardial paracentesis may be performed, although thoracotomy may also be done either from the outset or after paracentesis if the tamponade recurs.

Injuries to the heart and great vessels occur from time to time and are not invariably fatal as one might think. Massive volume replacement and very rapid thoracotomy are, however, the patient's only chance of survival.

HEAD INJURIES

When the patient arrives in the department the first concern is for resuscitation as detailed in Chapter 2. This will usually consist of airway care and the importance of this cannot be over-stated. An obstructed airway causes cerebral oedema which can increase rapidly. It will also worsen any pre-existing intracranial haemorrhage. As with all major injuries an i.v. cannula such as a Venflon should be inserted so that you have immediate access to a vein in an emergency.

Most head wounds can be treated fairly easily, simple pressure stopping the majority of bleeding. The hair round the wound will need to be shaved so that the wound is easily seen and ready for suturing later. Do not try to stop any bleeding from the inside of the ear, simply place a sterile pad over it to mop up the blood.

Despite what many nurses think, emergency surgical intervention is very rarely necessary with head injuries. In the majority of cases conservative management with very close observation for signs of raised intracranial pressure is all that is required.

Following a blow to the head, the brain can be compressed in three main ways:

- Bone can press onto the brain (depressed fracture)
- The brain itself can swell (cerebral oedema)
- Bleeding can occur inside the skull (extra, subdural or intracerebral haemorrhage)

It is essential that these complications are discovered quickly because, especially with the latter, permanent brain damage and death can quickly ensue.

Mannitol, steroids and hyperventilation have all been used following head injury to lower a raised intracranial pressure caused by cerebral oedema. For extra or subdural haemorrhages urgent burr holes will be required, even in an outlying hospital if time does not allow the luxury of transfer to a neurosurgical unit.

Computer tomography (CT/CAT scan)

Since the first edition of this book, CT scanning has become far more frequently used for head injuries so I think that it is now essential to go into a little detail about it.

The CT scanner is shown in Fig. 41. For your needs it is not necessary for you to have a knowledge of exactly how it works, suffice it to say that it takes x-ray 'slices' at any level through the patient's head. As well as showing up the bones as with normal x-rays it will also show up different densities of tissues and fluids (Fig. 42).

Usually a series of 'slices' are taken at different levels in the horizontal plane. The time taken for each slice varies with the machine used, from about three seconds to a minute, so, the whole process can take about 20 minutes. During this time the patient

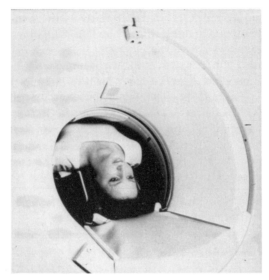

Fig. 41. *A CT scanner.* **(With kind permission of Siemans Ltd)**

must keep his head absolutely still. With many head injuries this will be impossible and a general anaesthetic will be required to ensure a clear run of pictures. If the patient is still conscious the procedure must be explained to him, both so that full cooperation can be obtained and for his own peace of mind that the gigantic and frightening machine will not cause pain.

Ensure that metal objects near patients' heads (i.e. hair clips, ear-rings, false teeth, safety pins, etc.) are removed and that if an

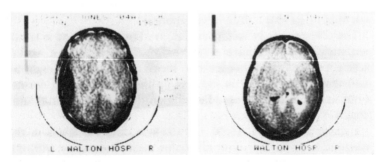

Fig. 42. A, *A CT scan showing an extradural haemorrhage on the patient's left side;* **B,** *A CT scan showing cerebral oedema with the ventricles displaced.*

endotracheal tube is in position, that it has plastic connections and the tubing is directed away from the head.

If you are required to stay with the patient, you will have to wear a lead apron while the scan is being done.

Even in units which have a CT scanner, not all the head injury patients have one done. This would be unnecessarily wasteful. Rather, the criteria used for deciding whether to take a scan are (a) where a skull fracture has been found (because intracranial haemorrhage is far more likely to occur in these patients) and (b) where there is an altered state of consciousness.

In outlying hospitals it is more likely to be used only when the patient's condition is causing 'concern'.

The CT scan will not mean that the patient will not require an ordinary x-ray. Bony deformity does show on the scan but not nearly as clearly as with ordinary film.

Do not get the false impression from all that has been written on complex examinations that every patient must go through this 'mill' before reverting to theatre. Nothing could be further from the truth. With a rapidly expanding extradural haemorrhage, as with many major trauma victims, the x-ray department is the last place that you want your patient.

Nursing observations

It is mainly by the charting of our head injury observations that the doctor will get a true impression of the progress of the patient's condition, telling him if the patient is developing raised intracranial pressure. The charts upkeep is essential, no matter how busy you are. Their frequency depends to a large extent on the patient's condition. For example, with a fully conscious, alert patient, every half to one hour may be satisfactory at the sister's discretion. But, with the unconscious or 'drowsy' every 10 to 15 minutes would be more appropriate.

All head injuries should be charted within minutes of arrival in a unit, so that a base-line is obtained on which other readings can be judged. The chart which is used (Fig. 43) should by now be fairly standardized throughout the country and is based on the Glasgow coma scale. This measures the patient's best verbal and motor response plus eye opening. Its use cuts down some of the mistakes that can occur between one member of staff and another, by the

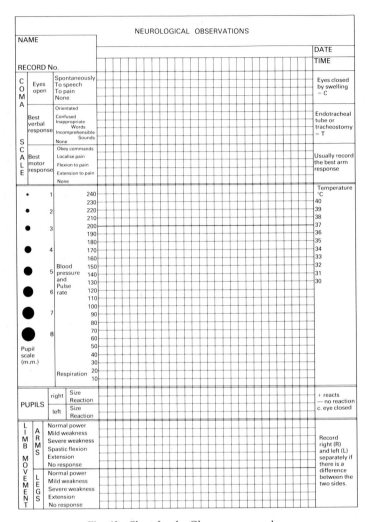

Fig. 43. *Chart for the Glasgow coma scale.*

standardization of terms. Confusion can still occur, especially when different forms of pain are used for initiating the motor response. The ideal is pressure on the fingernail with a pen. Other common problems arise with junior nurses not understanding what flexion and extension to pain means. It can take a little time for these to be seen on the department by a new staff nurse.

A final safeguard is for the same nurse to stay with the patient until arrival on the ward.

Examining the pupils. Many nurses worry about changes which can occur in the eyes following a head injury and consider that they are the 'be all and end all' of head injury observations. Of course pupil changes are important, but we should not get it out of perspective: *the lowering of the patient's level of consciousness is the most important factor for you to report.* Pupil changes can be difficult, even for the accident and emergency sister to interpret. Therefore, I shall say this. Tell sister of any change in the patient's pupil size, equality or reaction to light, so that she can assess the matter.

If a light is shone into an eye, the pupil should contract until the light source is removed. If this occurs, we say that the pupil 'reacts to light'. Unless there is previous disease, both pupils should be the same size. With raised intracranial pressure, after an initial period of contraction, the pupil on the affected side will steadily dilate and not react to light. The same sequence of events will also soon occur on the other side until both pupils become fixed and dilated.

Finally, but just as important as the above observations. When we consider an injured patient, we must think of him as a whole. Certainly, the head injury may be the most important injury present, but, as an accident and emergency nurse you must realize that you see before you a patient who has suffered a certain trauma. The main condition may seem to be a head injury, but he may have other injuries which you must look for now and be constantly on the alert for while he is with you.

FURTHER READING

Beeston, H. & Webber, E.G. (1983) Head injuries. *Nursing*, 2:15 (July), 442–444.
Goodison, S.M. (1982) Shock. *Nursing*, 1:33 (January), 1440–1442.
Guthrie, M.M. (Ed.) (1982) *Shock* (Contemporary Issues in Critical Care). Edinburgh: Churchill Livingstone.
Hayward, R. (1980) *Mangement of acute head injuries*. Oxford: Blackwell.
Huckstep, R.L. (1978) *A simple guide to trauma*, 2nd edn. Edinburgh: Churchill Livingstone.
Jennett, B. & Teasdale, G. (1981) *Management of head injuries*, 1st edn. Philadelphia: F.A. Davis & Co.

Keen, G. (1975) *Chest injuries*. Bristol: John Wright & Sons.
Odling-Smee, W. & Crockard, A. (1981) *Trauma care*, 1st edn. London: Academic Press.
Pearson, O.R. & Austin, R.T. (1979) *Accident surgery and orthopaedics for students*, 2nd edn. Chapters 8 and 9. London: Lloyd-Luke.

4 Care of major medical emergencies

To members of the public the word 'collapse' may denote anything from a simple faint to a cardiac arrest. Tactful and detailed questioning is often required to find out exactly what has happened. However, the collapsed patient forms a substantial part of the work load of an accident and emergency unit and such cases can be of immense interest. In many instances caring for such patients can be compared to fitting together the pieces of a diagnostic jigsaw, except that this has to be done 'against the clock'. You will find that well over 90 per cent of the patients that you will see fit easily into one of the categories described below.

DIABETES MELLITUS

As you all know, the control of diabetes depends on a very careful balance between insulin and the amount of carbohydrate which the patient takes in. The majority of diabetics cope very well with their disease, but, even the most careful make the occasional mistake or have a sudden illness which upsets the balance. That is when the accident and emergency department sees the patient. There are two specific conditions which can befall the patient:

1. Hypoglycaemia (hypo)
2. Ketoacidosis

Both conditions usually affect known diabetics; however, ketoacidosis is also sometimes seen when the patient first presents with the disease. Almost every diabetic patient you will have to care for on an accident and emergency unit will be 'hypo'; the ketoacidotic patient is comparatively uncommon.

Hypoglycaemia

The presentation of hypoglycaemia varies tremendously. Some patients arrive fully awake, just telling you that they are diabetics

and can feel themselves beginning to go 'off'. Others are staggering, confused, speaking incoherently and easily mistaken for
drunks. Lastly, and very commonly, patients may arrive deeply
unconscious. People accompanying the patient will speak of the
fairly rapid onset of the signs and symptoms and will also, on
deeper questioning, reveal that the patient may have missed a
meal.

If the patient is unconscious, specific things to look for include:

1. Profuse sweating, sometimes to such an extent that the
   clothing is literally saturated
2. Tachycardia
3. Injection marks on the thighs, abdomen or arm
4. A diabetic card in the pocket or a Medic-Alert bracelet or
   medallion (Fig. 44)
5. Sweets or sugar

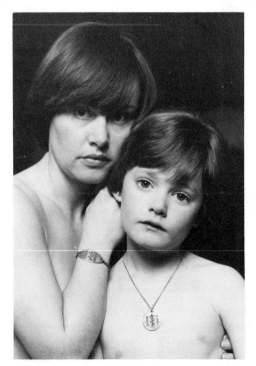

Fig. 44. *A Medic-Alert bracelet or medallion can warn of any condition from which
the wearer suffers.* (**With kind permission of Medic-Alert Foundation**)

Initial care

While the patient is being undressed and examined, a reagent test strip for glucose in the blood, such as Dextrostix or B.M. Stix, is taken to give a rough idea of the patient's blood sugar level. The doctor will then take a specimen of blood to send off for an accurate blood sugar estimation. If the patient is awake and still able to cooperate with you, sweet drinks are all that are required. About 20 g of dextrose monohydrate in a glass of milk will still be fairly palatable for the patient and will give about three 'black lines' (one 'black line' = 10 g carbohydrate). This may be followed by intravenous therapy depending on the patient's response. If the patient is unconscious, the very first essential is the care of the airway as mentioned in Chapter 2. For drugs the intravenous route has to be used. Fifty millilitres of 50% Dextrose is usually given and in most circumstances will bring about a dramatic improvement. The patient often wakes up and starts to talk while the needle is still in situ, just as in the Hollywood movies! While this intravenous dextrose is being given you are often faced with an extremely restless patient who is rolling over and fighting your every move. Several nurses must be available to help restrain the patient otherwise the doctor's task will be impossible. If an i.v. injection is impossible, one unit of glucagon, i.m., can be given and repeated after 20 minutes.

Once your patient has fully recovered he will not necessarily have to stay in hospital. Indeed, most diabetics from time to time suffer such attacks, usually in the milder form, and when relieved continue with their daily routine. However, always have the patient accompanied home. One final point, a severe hypoglycaemic coma is a medical emergency. If the blood sugar is very low for a prolonged period severe irreversible brain damage will occur; treatment, therefore, must be prompt.

Ketoacidosis

The ketoacidotic patient presents a very serious medical emergency, but, compared to the 'hypo', will be a comparative rarity. You will be able to notice certain features about such patients:

1. They are not necessarily unconscious, which is why I have not used the term 'diabetic coma'. They may vary from fully

awake, through varying degrees of semiconsciousness to a deep coma.
2. The onset of the condition will have been slow, over a day or days, in complete contrast to 'hypo' patients.
3. They will be dehydrated and may be shocked.
4. The skin will be dry and they may have air hunger. You may be able to notice on the breath a strange smell like nail varnish.
5. There may be an infection somewhere in the body.
6. There will be an excess of sugar in the urine and blood.

Treatment must be rapid and senior medical assistance should be sought from the outset. Your patient should not spend much time in the accident and emergency department; however, treatment may be commenced by you as follows. If the patient is unconscious, the airway must be your prime consideration. Blood specimens will need to be sent to the laboratory for estimation of sugar, electrolytes and blood gases. Soluble insulin will be administered intravenously and/or intramuscularly. An intravenous infusion will be set up, to administer 0.9% sodium chloride. A potassium supplement may also be required. Depending on the patient's condition a nasogastric tube and catheter may be introduced in the department. This may be followed by an infusion of 5% Dextrose (154 mmol/litre). During the patient's transfer to the ward, remember that vomiting occurs frequently with this condition and be prepared.

CONVULSIONS

The diagnosis of a 'fit' is usually straight forward, especially if it occurs in the accident and emergency department. Most, however, occur outside, sometimes even without an audience. By the time the patient is found he is just lying still or acting strangely. When this occurs the nurse has to help the doctor gather together the information so that the correct diagnosis can be reached. Notice pointers such as:

1. The patient still in a deep sleep
2. The patient acting and speaking strangely
3. The patient may not know what has happened and be disorientated

4. Injuries, especially grazes round the face
5. A painful or lacerated tongue
6. Incontinence
7. Tablets or a card in the pocket

It is sad, but the stigma of epilepsy is still with us today. When talking to your patients you will find that many will admit to having fits, blackouts, dizzy spells or 'turns', but not many come forward and say 'I have epilepsy'. This alone can produce problems and, when added to the mental confusion when the patient first wakes up, can put the diagnosis in doubt for an hour or more until a relative arrives to give a correct history. Even with a known epileptic who does not appear to have hurt himself, have him lying down on a trolley with cot sides raised. The patient should be undressed so that the doctor can examine thoroughly; it is surprising how many small injuries can be found which the patient did not notice at first. Epileptics are also just as likely as any other person to have had a coronary thrombosis, cerebrovascular accident, subdural haematoma and the like, and the doctor will want to exclude such other conditions first. A head injury chart may need to be commenced.

If you are with the patient as he has a fit, you must observe it carefully and give the doctor an accurate description. Notice the following:

1. Any loss of consciousness
2. Was the fit generalized?
3. Did it start in one part of the body and then spread?
4. How long did it last?

The family of an epileptic will become distressed if the patient does not return home on time. Therefore, as soon as is practicable, send a message to the relatives so that they will know what has occurred. The majority will be very thankful that the patient is in safe hands and even offer to take him home if they have transport.

Care during a 'fit'

If your patient is having a 'fit', first of all ensure that he is secure on the accident trolley with the sides firmly up. Try to prevent the tongue from being trapped between the teeth, but if it is trapped and the fitting is prolonged, attempt to ease it free using padded spatulas or a gag. Do this extremely gently and if the tongue is free leave the teeth alone. Use suction to remove any froth from the mouth. Do not be too alarmed by the cyanosis of the tonic phase. This is caused by the respiratory muscles being in spasm and will revert to normal after about 30 seconds as long as all the rules for care of the airway, as mentioned in Chapter 2, are observed. During the clonic phase, ensure that limbs and head do not bang against the trolley sides, but otherwise there is no need to restrain the patient in any way.

Lastly, stay with the patient until he has fully recovered, ensure privacy and explain what has happened. Help may be needed if the patient has been incontinent. The patient will probably want to sleep for a while and later get dressed and have a drink before going home. Never let the patient leave the department unaccompanied because of the dangers of another fit or of post-epileptic automatism.

Diazepam may be asked for and may help to prevent further fits occurring. In many instances the fit has been caused by alteration in either the patient's drugs or the doses and advice may be needed about them.

Status epilepticus

Status epilepticus, a state of continuous fitting, is a serious condition which will be fatal if allowed to continue for very long. Apart from constant care of the airway and oxygen administration, an intravenous infusion will have to be set up. Drugs such as paraldehyde, diazepam and chlormethiazole may be used.

CHEST PAIN

Patients who present themselves at the accident and emergency department with chest pain may have anything from the trivial muscular ache to an aortic aneurysm. A strict routine has to be adopted to ensure that no patient with a severe condition slips through the 'net'. Never keep a patient with chest pain waiting, however busy you are; always err on the side of safety and let them 'jump the queue'.

The pain associated with an acute myocardial infarction is not always as described in textbooks, indeed sometimes there is no pain at all. For safety, always presume the patient has had an acute myocardial infarction until the doctor has reached a diagnosis. This condition is about the most unpredictable I have ever come across. I have seen the worst patient rally round and pull through *but* I have also been speaking to young patients with previously normal ECGs who have 'arrested' in front of me. The youngest patient I have ever known to die of acute myocardial infarction was only 21 years old and previously a very fit football player. I am sure that this is not a record. Never forget its *unpredictability*.

The nursing routine to be adopted is:

1. Put the patient on a trolley, near to resuscitation equipment
2. If the patient seems very ill, take off clothing above the waist; if apparently well the patient can be completely undressed
3. The patient should be in the position which he finds most comfortable
4. Take the temperature, pulse, respiration and blood pressure
5. An ECG should be taken
6. If an acute myocardial infarction is diagnosed, attach the chest electrodes and place the patient on a monitor
7. Stay with or near the patient
8. Never let any of the urgency of the situation, consciously or unconsciously, be passed on to the patient. There should always be a prevailing atmosphere of relaxation and calm to allay the patient's worries

A fairly standard medical regimen for an acute myocardial infarction might be as follows:

1. Insertion of a Venflon intravenous cannula.
2. Oxygen by MC or similar mask
3. Diamorphine hydrochloride for pain and rest (intravenous and/or intramuscular)
4. Prochlorperazine to prevent vomiting

Always explain to your patient why the treatments are being done; do not lie, but 'play down' the reasons.

Transiderm-nitro. This is a comparatively new product on the market which I think you should know about. It is basically glyceryl trinitrate on the pad of a plaster which is stuck to the chest wall. I give it particular mention firstly because in the future it may gain popularity and secondly so that if you see a patient with such a plaster you will know that they suffer from ischaemic heart disease and will therefore have a hint to a diagnosis. The 'plaster' is renewed every 24 hours and placed on a fresh area of skin.

Electrocardiograph and monitor

Electrocardiograph. It is important that the specialist accident and emergency nurse is able to take a full 12-lead ECG; not that it should necessarily be a routine 'job', but that she should be able to do it if circumstances or the convenience of the patient warrant it. After being some time on the unit she should also know the *basis* of its interpretation and be able to 'see' an obvious acute myocardial infarction. She should know how to get a clear 'picture' on the monitor and be able to recognize some of the main arrhythmias. It is beyond the scope of this book to delve into this subject too deeply. However, below are a few hints on taking ECGs and fault-finding.

Explain what you are about to do and that the patient will feel no pain. An ECG machine with all its leads can appear to be monstrous to those who have never seen one before. The patient should be lying comfortably with arms at the sides and not touching the cot sides. Ask him to lie as still as possible; even small movements, shivering or a cough can make the trace poor.

Before the limb electrodes are attached rub a little of the electrode jelly into the skin; this will aid conductivity. Ensure that all the connections are firm, at the patient and at the machine end. A loose connection can give you an apparently dead patient which can be rather unnerving.

The position of the chest electrodes is shown in Fig. 45. Difficulty may be encountered if the patient has a hairy chest, the sucker failing before the trace has been completed. This is easily overcome without shaving, simply smooth all the hair away from the central position.

Three faults occur commonly on a tracing (Fig. 46). The first is a distorted base-line caused by the patient moving or the muscles twitching. In the second the base-line appears as a wide band; this

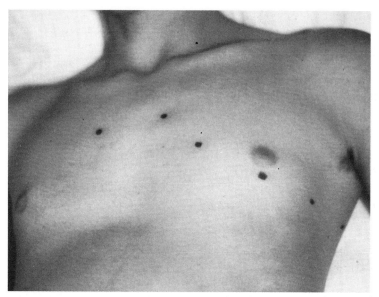

Fig. 45. *The position of the six chest electrodes used when taking an electrocardiogram.*

is caused by electrical interference. Try changing the socket into which the machine is plugged or turning off nearby electrical apparatus. Thirdly, a base-line which wanders all over the paper usually occurs in a restless patient. Either do a trace in the moments when he is still or coax the patient to relax more and go 'limp'.

A minimum of three complexes is required for each lead, but try not to go to the other extreme finishing up with yards of streamer. A badly taken ECG is worse than none at all; persuade an expert to teach you so that you can produce tracings of quality.

Monitor. Much of what has already been said applies also to the monitor. Unlike the ECG, the monitor is only there to help diagnose cardiac arrhythmias. Three of these have already been mentioned in Chapter 2, that is ventricular fibrillation, asystole and ventricular standstill. Although there are many, I now wish to mention just one more; ventricular extrasystoles (ectopics) (Fig. 47). Although even healthy people can have ectopics from time to

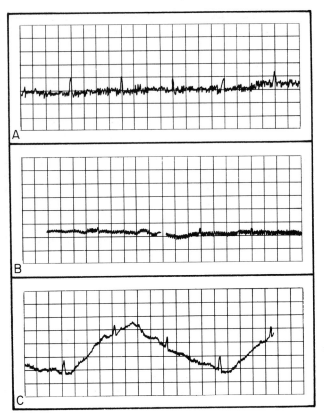

Fig. 46. *Three common faults in taking an ECG: **A**, distorted base-line caused by the patient moving or by his muscles twitching; **B**, a wide base-line caused by electrical interference; and **C**, a wandering base-line caused by the patient moving.*

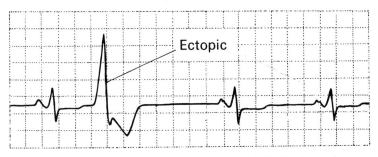

Fig. 47. *Ventricular ectopic beats. The patient died shortly afterwards.*

time, they are of special significance following an acute myocardial infarction. Cardiac arrest may be imminent in any of the following circumstances:

1. If more than six ectopics occur in a minute
2. If they occur in runs (salvos)
3. If they are multi-focal (have different shapes)
4. If they occur on or near the preceding T wave

A thorough understanding of the cardiac monitor makes your work far more interesting and adds to your usefulness as a nurse. Nursing knowledge must keep pace with medical progress. A patient with a cardiac disorder has a basic right to be cared for by someone with specialized knowledge, who can recognize the approach of disaster and not just sit waiting to see if it arrives. Further excellent reading on the subject is mentioned at the end of the chapter.

CEREBROVASCULAR ACCIDENT

To wake up and want to speak and yet be unable to make the words; to want to touch and yet be unable to move: the frustrations and fear of a patient with a cerebrovascular accident must be immense. We must do our utmost to allay the patient's fears, explain simply what has happened and give encouragement for the future, both to the patient and to the relatives.

With this group of patients, diagnosis is comparatively easy for the doctor, and for the nurse the care is that of any unconscious patient. However, I do want to make a special mention here of patients with a subarachnoid haemorrhage. This usually occurs in a younger age group than the usual 'stroke' patient and even children can be affected. The commonest cause is the rupture of a small 'berry' aneurysm at the base of the brain, which in many instances can be surgically treated with excellent results.

The patient may or may not be unconscious and the following occur:

1. Neck stiffness
2. Severe occipital headaches (relatives may say the patient had these beforehand)
3. Intense vomiting

4. Confusion, drowsiness, coma
5. Lumbar puncture shows blood in the cerebrospinal fluid

THE BREATHLESS PATIENT

Of the many medical causes of acute breathlessness seen in the accident and emergency department, the majority will fall into these four groups:

1. Exacerbation of chronic bronchitis
2. Bronchial asthma
3. Pneumonia
4. Acute left ventricular failure

The care that we as nurses give to all of the patients is similar. Firstly, they should be sat up. Some will only be able to tolerate sitting sideways on the trolley with their legs dangling over the side. Although this at first seems unorthodox, if it makes the patient more comfortable it is best. For some who are 'respiratory cripples', the ambulance journey will have been so exhausting that they will not even want to be lifted over onto the trolley. This may continue perhaps for many minutes until they have caught up with the 'oxygen deficit'. Let your patients once again be your guide, they know far more about their capabilities than you do. An opened window is another frequent request, giving your patient a sense of freedom.

A preliminary measurement of temperature, pulse, respiration and blood pressure is required and at some stage an ECG will be ordered. The doctor will in most instances have time for a fairly thorough examination of the chest before any treatment is commenced.

A chest radiograph is obviously required, but this is usually done after initial treatment or when the patient is on the way to the ward. It may show, for instance, the consolidation of pneumonia, a pneumothorax or the mottling of pulmonary oedema. It is best to have the patient accompanied by a nurse all the time in the x-ray department, firstly for reassurance and comfort of the patient, and also in case of deterioration which can occasionally be rapid. A spontaneous pneumothorax, i.e. one that occurs without preceding trauma, is a fairly common occurrence. It is seen especially in young, tall, thin people and those with previous chest conditions such as asthma or emphysema.

Presenting as chest pain and breathlessness of sudden onset, the patient will in most instances require the insertion of a chest drain. Blood gas analysis may be required; the sample is usually taken from the femoral artery in a heparinized syringe.

With asthmatic patients, beware of those with a severe tachycardia or an irregular pulse: they are very ill and sudden death can occur. Seek senior medical assistance immediately.

In the last few years the initial treatment of patients with acute bronchial asthma has changed significantly. Most now are given considerable relief by inhaling a mixture of salbutamol (Ventolin) and water in a nebulizer worked from the ordinary wall oxygen. A typical dose might be 1 ml of salbutamol nebulizer solution mixed with 4 ml water. The nebulizer produces a fine drenching mist which 'reaches the parts other beers cannot' and quite remarkably eases the bronchospasm often within minutes (Fig. 48).

Oxygen therapy

In most instances of breathlessness controlled oxygen therapy will be required. This can, and in some cases *must*, be given to the patient before the arrival of the doctor. No harm will come to the patient as long as the correct concentrations are given.

Two types of mask are available:

1. One which gives a high concentration of oxygen, for example, the MC mask giving 60% at 8 litres/minute.
2. One which gives a low concentration of oxygen, for example, the Ventimask, which can give varying concentrations accurately: 24, 28, 35, 38%.

As a general rule, but by no means in every instance, the following will apply until the doctor arrives. For the patient with chronic bronchitis, give a low percentage of oxygen, i.e. 24%, to start off with. For a patient with pneumonia, give 60% oxygen. For acute left ventricular failure give 60% oxygen. For acute bronchial asthma, start off at 24% oxygen. With all of these, bear in mind that we cannot accurately diagnose our patients' ills. So if they deteriorate the oxygen may have to be altered.

*

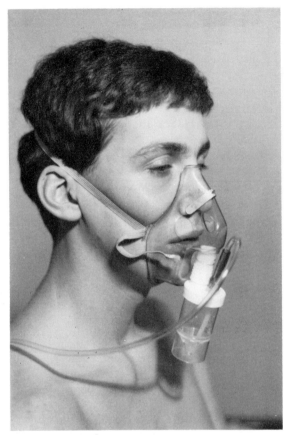

Fig. 48. *Salbutamol being used as a nebulizer.*

Drugs which may have to be given are listed in Table 2.

HAEMATEMESIS AND MELAENA

Mention has already been made in Chapter 3 of severe haemorrhage, but a few extra points are worthy of note on this topic. Firstly, always consider gastrointestinal haemorrhage a possibility in any patient who has fainted or 'collapsed' for no apparent reason and remains pale. Next, remember that blood from the stomach may be a brown colour, classically called 'coffee-

Table 2. *Drugs given for certain chest conditions.*

Condition	Drug (dose)
Asthma	Aminophylline (250 mg approx.) Hydrocortisone (100 mg)
Acute left ventricular failure	Frusemide (40 mg) Diamorphine hydrochloride (5 mg) Aminophylline (250 mg approx.)
Chronic bronchitis	Aminophylline (250 mg approx.)

grounds'. In most cases the stools will be black and tarry, and a rectal examination should be suggested to determine this. Beware of the black stool of patients taking iron supplements, though. Patients are not always forthcoming with information such as the colour of vomit or faeces and this has to be asked for. The vomiting of fresh blood is particularly frightening for the patient (and a junior nurse), so send a senior nurse to the ward with the patient. The nurse's confidence and ability can thus filter through to the patient.

ANAPHYLACTIC SHOCK

This is a devastating condition which is fairly uncommon and is caused by the body having a severe reaction to a foreign substance. The most frequent causes are penicillin, vaccines and stings.

The reaction starts almost immediately with urticaria, swelling of the air passages, severe bronchospasm and profound shock. Treatment must be immediate with intravenous injections of adrenaline, chlorpheniramine and hydrocortisone, if the patient's life is to be saved.

Only this year a patient in his thirties died before he arrived at our accident and emergency department, following an injection of penicillin.

FURTHER READING

Hubner, P.J.B. (1980) *Nurses' guide to cardiac monitoring*, 3rd edn. London: Baillière Tindall.

Rutherford, W. *et al* (1980) *Accident and emergency medicine*, 1st edn. London: Pitman Medical.

Sahn, S. A. (1983) *Pulmonary emergencies*. Edinburgh: Churchill Livingstone.

Smith, M. (1982) Respiratory emergencies. *Nursing Mirror*, 154 (March) Clinical Forum, 3:ii–iv, vi.

Watkins, P.J. (1982) ABC of diabetes. Diabetic emergencies. *British Medical Journal*, 285: 31 (July), 360–363.

5 Obstetric and gynaecological emergencies

RUPTURED ECTOPIC PREGNANCY

The diagnosis of ruptured ectopic pregnancy should be borne in mind with any female patient of child-bearing age presenting with abdominal pain. Your questioning of the patient, even if young or unmarried, should always include 'When was your last period?'. On occasions, the haemorrhage can be torrential, the patient arriving exsanguinated. Massive volume replacement may be required followed by urgent transfer to theatre.

BLEEDING IN EARLY PREGNANCY

Although the majority of patients with bleeding in early pregnancy will be 'direct admissions' to the wards, now and again they come of their own accord to the accident and emergency department for help. Whatever 'group' they belong to, all should be briefly assessed by a nurse as soon as possible after arrival because haemorrhage can sometimes be severe, even in a patient who walks in.

It is far kinder to the patient if the initial examination by a doctor is done routinely by the gynaecologist on call, rather than the patient having to be seen first by the casualty officer.

The following care may be required for a patient with an inevitable abortion:

- An analgesic (e.g. pethidine)
- Monitoring of the pulse, blood pressure and vaginal loss
- Blood may be taken for grouping and cross-matching
- An i.v. infusion may be commenced
- Oxytocic drugs
- Any vaginal discharge or clots should be saved for the doctor to examine
- Remember to allay the patient's anxiety about soiling their

clothes or the hospital sheets; many are extremely embarrassed

- It must be stressed that this is an extremely disturbing time for both the patient and her husband; their hopes of parenthood being quashed, possibly not for the first time. Throughout their stay in the department both will require explanation, reassurance and comfort. To us as nurses an inevitable abortion can seem so ordinary, commonplace and simple to deal with, that it is easy to forget the profound upset which it can cause.

RAPE VICTIMS

In most instances, cases of rape in this country go directly to the local police station where they are examined by the police surgeon with the aid of a policewoman. Although they will try to be as kind as possible, the very nature of the building itself will not help to calm the patient.

Fairly recently, moves have been made towards having such patients examined in hospitals, once again by the police surgeon but with a nurse present to assist him. It is obvious that such a clinical environment and the presence of a nurse would be of immense benefit to the patient making her feel that she is in a far more cherished, helping position. Although it is only likely to occur slowly, the accident and emergency nurse should be prepared for such cases to become more common and bear in mind a few simple points:

- The patient and even her clothing must be left undisturbed until the police surgeon arrives.
- Ensure absolute privacy for the patient, in a separate room.
- The patient, who will probably be severely distressed, will need all the psychological help you can give by staying with her, explaining to her about the doctor's examination and being generally reassuring.

The above comments relate to patients who have no other serious injuries. If on the other hand, the casualty officer has to intervene because of the patient's other injuries, as little disturbance as possible is to be made to the clothing. Any which is removed should be placed in a plastic bag. If possible no cleaning should be done round the thighs, groins, perineum or abdomen until the patient has been seen by the police surgeon.

IMMINENT CHILDBIRTH

Childbirth is a rarity to most accident and emergency departments, firstly because the ambulance service take most cases directly to the maternity department and secondly those who have their own transport usually know exactly where to go. However, sometimes people get lost and end up on our doorstep and sometimes, believe it or not, some just do not realize that they are pregnant until just before the birth (I have seen a few over the years). The other group of patients who can mistakenly arrive in the department are those who think they are having an abortion and finish up having a live birth. A foetus is said to be viable after about the 20th week of the pregnancy.

Patient care

While waiting for the obstetrician or midwife to arrive position your patient comfortably on her back with absorbent padding material under the buttocks. It is to be hoped that the department has had the foresight to have a sterile delivery pack made up for such occurrences. This should be opened by a runner nurse while you quickly scrub up and put on a mask, cap and gown. Remember that the pregnancy is not happening routinely, the patient will often be anxious even if she has had children before. So, it is up to you, the nurse, to calm the patient down by your very actions and words. Remember you want an air of calm, efficiency and privacy to settle the mother. Interested participants and spectators must be diverted elsewhere.

Encourage the patient to hold her breath and push down during the contractions and to relax between them. Do your best to have at least cleaned the perineum and covered the anus over with sterile gauze. Place sterile towels between her legs and over the abdomen. Support the baby's head with your gloved hand as it emerges, ensuring that it's journey is smooth and controlled and that there is no cord round the neck. As soon as possible clean secretions away from the baby's face and suck out the mouth with a mucus extractor.

After the baby has been delivered, the cord can be clamped in two places and then cut. Wrap the baby up to minimize heat loss and give it to the mother.

By this time it is hoped that knowledgeable assistance has arrived and you can have a well-earned cup of tea. If not, round two will follow shortly with the passing of the placenta. Do not pull on the cord to help it out. Save the placenta so that it can be examined by the midwife to ensure that it is intact and healthy.

FURTHER READING

Cohen, A. W. (1981) *Emergencies in obstetrics and gynaecology*. Edinburgh: Churchill Livingstone.

Shorthouse, M.A. & Brush, M.G. (1981) *Gynaecology in nursing practice*. London: Baillière Tindall.

6 Soft tissue injuries

To people in some occupations a 2 cm wound on the hand can be as incapacitating, physically and financially, as a fractured leg to you or me. To a child, a drop of blood can appear a horrific torrent. Buried glass and damage to tendons, nerves or even a major artery can go unnoticed by the unwary.

When dealing with wounds the first priority is, of course, to deal with torrential haemorrhage, which has already been described in a previous chapter. Let us now start at the beginning and consider all the other aspects of care.

The patient

To some people the sight of blood is terrifying, especially if it is their own. Patients react very differently to injuries. For instance, a tiny child with a horrific wound may be as 'good as gold' and settle easily, whereas a huge labourer may be as 'white as a sheet' following a minute finger injury. The lesson to be learned is, therefore, never to have a trolley too far away, since you never know when your patient may require it. Always reassure the patient by your actions and words.

It is humorous indeed to see some of the first-aid dressings used by members of the public: huge bath towels engulfing the patient, also nylon stockings or socks tied round the limbs to act as tourniquets (Fig. 49).

If a patient arrives with a blood-soaked bandage around even a fairly minor wound, he or she should be seen by a nurse within a few minutes to allay any worries. He or she can assess the seriousness of the wound and place a temporary dressing on it. It will then be a far more contented patient who waits, perhaps an hour or more, to see the doctor.

Aseptic technique

The state of wounds on an accident and emergency department must not be likened to anything you will see on a ward. They are as different as chalk and cheese. They must be treated differently if

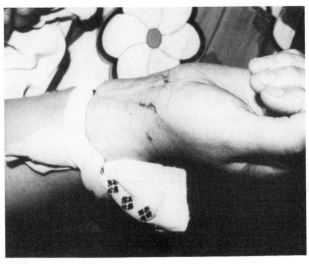

Fig. 49. *Many members of the public still believe that a tourniquet like this is essential. Take every opportunity of forbidding their routine use.*

they are to heal successfully. They are compared in Table 3.

The whole question of aseptic technique on an accident and emergency department requires appraisal. We must not pretend that using forceps, donning a mask and gently swabbing a wound are going to do much to save our patients from wound infection. In theory, the wearing of a mask and using forceps whilst doing dressings should lessen the contamination of the wound. In

Table 3. *Types of wound*

Ward wound	Accident and emergency wound
Caused by a sterile scalpel	Caused by a contaminated object
Made in the theatre	Made in dirty surroundings
Tissues almost always healthy	Often contains dead or devitalized tissue
Skin very clean	Skin dirty
Hardly ever contaminated	Always contaminated
Usually incised	Usually jagged

practice, however, on an accident and emergency department this is not borne out. Under standard accident conditions, the wearing of a mask is a pointless pretence. Forceps will sometimes hinder your cleaning and not be as gentle as a hand, whereas cheap and clean polythene gloves are ideal. What *will* cut down the number of infected wounds and be many times more effective than a full aseptic technique is the following initial treatment:

1. Thorough cleaning of the surrounding skin
2. Thorough mechanical cleaning of the wound. Use sterile swabs soaked in an antiseptic solution such as chlorhexidine and cetrimide (Savlon) and held with your fingers

These two essentials will do more to protect your patient than any other ward-oriented method. With this in mind, the following approach must be made if a consistently high success rate is to be achieved.

Cleaning the surrounding skin. As an example of skin cleansing let us consider a lacerated hand. First, forget the wound and concentrate on the surrounding skin. On a large scale, this can mean a miner being thoroughly washed from head to toe. On a smaller scale it can mean a garage mechanic or farmer having *both* arms thoroughly cleaned with soap and water. For the ordinary man in the street, it can mean washing off minimal dirt from the whole hand. While this is being done, a large wound can be protected by gauze packed in it. With small cuts, on the finger, for example, this is impracticable. With wounds of the fingers or toes simply dip the whole hand or foot into the water to get it clean. Children can be coaxed to 'play' in the water once they find that it will not sting. Instead of just rubbing the hand to get the dirt off it can easily be made into a child's game.

Cleaning the wound itself. Small particles of grit can be picked out of the wound using plain McIndoe's forceps or splinter forceps. The plastic type of forceps seen in most packs these days is useless for this task. Hydrogen peroxide also has a good mechanical action, 'bubbling' furiously when in contact with open flesh and therefore loosening dirt. Warn your patient, however, of its burning sensation.

Gauze tends to be more abrasive than cotton wool, so is far better at removing ingrained dirt. Cotton wool also has the disadvantage of leaving threads on the wound, especially if it is used for drying.

Although gentleness is of the utmost importance, let us not forget our first aim, that of thorough cleaning of the wound. If dirt is embedded you have to rub to get it out, even if this hurts the patient. A little pain initially will perhaps prevent an infected wound later.

The cleaning of filthy grazes, seen extensively with motor cyclists, can be achieved with far less discomfort for the patient if a 10% lignocaine (Xylocaine) spray is applied first and then the rubbing is done after about three to four minutes with a sterile brush.

Grazes of the face must be cleaned scrupulously so that permanent 'tattooing' does not occur. If tattooing is severe, toilet under local or general anaesthesia may be required.

To get oil or grease off the skin use Swarfega or similar grease solvent. This is smeared all over the affected skin and can even be rubbed into lacerations without doing any harm. If it then washed off with water after a few minutes.

Dispense with a ward idea of wiping a wound a single time with the swab in a particular direction. In these cases the whole field contains bacteria, rubbing can be in any direction and often the swab must be used like a toothbrush to remove dirt completely.

To many of you who are used to ward dressings, much of the above will be strange and against what you have been taught in the past. Balance this, however, with the completely different type of case seen and the fact that this method works in practice. Lastly, before the subject of aseptic technique is concluded, this technique is only for the initial reception of casualties. All the normal rules apply to other situations such as minor suturing, the accident and emergency theatre and dressings at a review clinic.

The closure of wounds

Steristrips. Adhesive strips are ideal to use in certain instances, but should not be used indiscriminately. There is a definite place for both Steristrips and suturing and care should be taken that adhesive strips do not become the 'lazy man's stitch'. The surrounding skin must be perfectly dry; several minutes may be required for this. With screaming, hot, perspiring children the task

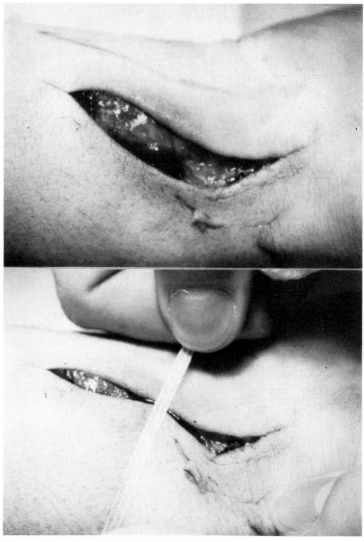

Fig. 50. *The edges of the wound are first brought together roughly so that the Steristrips can be positioned accurately.*

is difficult. To overcome this some use Tinct. Benzoin Co., but this can sting if it accidentally enters the wound. Strips with Tinct. Benzoin impregnated in the material may be advantageous. The edges of the wound are brought together (Fig. 50) but gaps must

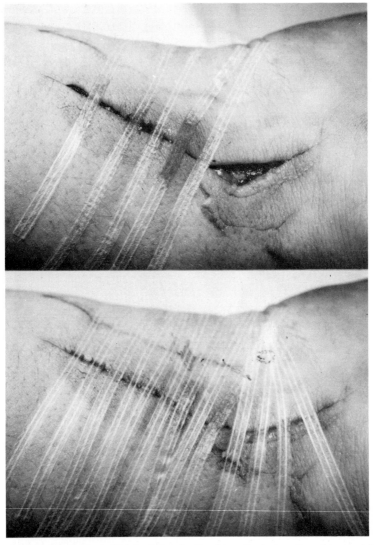

Fig. 51. *A laceration which healed well using 3 mm Steristrips. Note the essential gaps between each strip.*

be left between the Steristrips for the wound exudate to escape (Fig. 51). This is vital. As the strips are applied, some of the earlier ones may have to be removed because they have become slack. Continue until you get perfect apposition. For facial wounds, or other delicate work, use the 3 mm size and possibly cut these in half so that you can get an accurate pull in the desired direction. Steristrips can be used on the scalp; only a small area of hair requires shaving on either side of the wound, however to be successful this hair will have to be shaved close to the skin (i.e. no stubble left at all), otherwise the Steristrips will not stick. They are not suitable for skin which moves a lot, for example:

1. Finger-web spaces
2. The centre of the palm
3. Near or on the lips
4. Behind the knee

Steristrips can be used alongside sutures or alternatively internal catgut sutures can take up the tension of the wound and the surface can then be finished with Steristrips. Ensure that the strips stick right up to the edge of the wound. If not they may have the effect of inverting the wound edges (Fig. 52). This will delay healing and cause a scar. If you cannot get them to do the job correctly suggest suture.

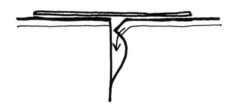

Fig. 52. *If the Steristrip does not stick right up to the edge of the wound, inversion of the non-stuck edge may occur.*

Basic wound suture. All the preliminary cleaning of the surrounding skin must be carried out as mentioned previously. The preparatory cleaning of the wound itself, however, can be just the minimum required to remove excess dirt. All the remaining cleaning and removal of dead tissue can be done after a local or general anaesthetic has been given. Full aseptic technique must be observed throughout the procedure.

The basic equipment pack is as follows:

Two towels
Gloves

Gauze swabs
Antiseptic
Needles, syringes and local anaesthetic
Suture material (for example, black silk or nylon)
Needle holder
Toothed dissecting forceps
Suture scissors
Dressing of Melolin or other non-stick dressing
Bandage

Prepare your patient by explaining what will happen. It is surprising how many patients, even adults, have simply no idea what awaits them and are scared. Never lie to your patient by saying 'It won't hurt', when it will; it is better to say it will hurt a little but play it down. Always have the patient lying down on a trolley, just in case of faintness. Children should have one parent sitting by their side all the time (if the parent is willing) to give comfort. Asking the parents to wait outside may be convenient for the nurse, but not for the patient.

Babies and toddlers are best wrapped up in a blanket or draw sheet to stop tiny arms and legs flying around in all directions. Protect the patients' clothing from further damage by blood, although in many instances they will tell you not to bother because it is ruined already. If injections for tetanus are required in children, wait until after the suturing is done before giving them. The doctor will then have a better chance of suturing on a settled and quiet patient.

Towelling can easily surround the wound if a hole is cut with scissors in the centre of a paper towel. Alternatively, the towel can be laid on one side of the wound nearest the operator. Never cover the face of a child completely; it will be frightening.

Lignocaine 1% plain is the local anaesthetic to use in most instances, although 2% is occasionally asked for. Lignocaine with adrenaline may also occasionally be asked for by the doctor, but should be kept separately under lock and key so that the two do not become mixed up. If lignocaine with adrenaline was to be injected accidentally into a finger, gangrene would be likely to occur. This is too great a risk to take. As well as checking yourself, always show the ampoule to the operator before the solution is drawn up to help to prevent mistakes. A 23G or 25G needle will be required for the injection; some prefer to use a dental syringe and needle so as to gain the added length available to such narrow gauges. The patient's pain is dependent on both the thickness of the needle and the amount of local injected. The skin is cleaned and then lignocaine is injected around the wound; the plunger of the syringe is withdrawn at intervals to ensure that injection is not being given intravenously. The operator must avoid the injection of excessive amounts of lignocaine which will distort the wound and further damage the tissues.

The suture material used can be very varied and is best dictated by the examining doctor. A fairly standard material is black silk, which should be available in sizes from 2/0, for a large wound where great strength is required, through to 6/0 which is very fine and used for very delicate work around the face and eyes. For the majority of wounds, which are on the hands and fingers, 3/0 and 4/0 are ideal. A variety of plain catgut should be on hand, both on its own and with needles; 2/0, 3/0 and 4/0 should be adequate for most needs. Dexon is used by many, especially in the smaller sizes, 4/0 and 5/0. It is used for suturing in places where removal of sutures would be difficult and painful for the patient. Nylon sutures are used in some centres.

Further details of how to perform a simple suture are given in Appendix IV.

Some miscellaneous aspects of wound care

The ring block. The ring block is used to anaesthetize the whole of a finger or toe. About 5 ml of lignocaine 1% or 2% are injected near to the digital nerve on either side of the base of the digit (Fig. 53).

Apart from injecting the wrong site, the most common mistake is to start suturing immediately after injection, instead of waiting five minutes or so for the injection to work.

'One quick stitch'. By 'one quick stitch' I mean not giving a local anaesthetic to children thinking that it will be 'kinder' when only one or two sutures are required.

Against this argument I wish to place the following facts:
1. One suture necessitates two pricks of the suture needle plus

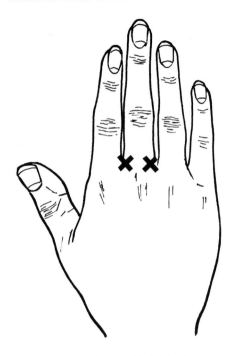

Fig. 53. *Sites for ring-block injections.*

the uncomfortable sensation of the thread being pulled through and tightened.

2. The skin will also sometimes have to be held by toothed forceps.
3. The suturing, which must be done accurately if scarring is to be prevented, is done on a struggling child. A delicate job cannot, therefore, be done.

Shins. The shin is indeed a perilous place for a wound, especially if the patient has rheumatoid arthritis or is taking steroids. The skin becomes as thin as tissue paper. Elderly ladies are particularly vulnerable. The blood supply to the skin of the shin is mainly in a longitudinal direction, so lacerations in particular directions can leave parts with a very poor blood supply (Fig. 54). The early help of a plastic surgeon for grafting can be advantageous. Skin closures such as Steristrips can be of great use here, enabling a hold to be

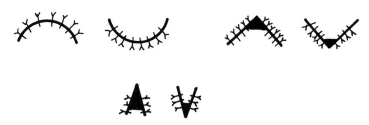

Fig. 54. *Lacerations to the shin. Shaded areas represent estimated necrosis of skin.*

kept on the skin where a suture would simply pull out as the knot is tightened.

Glass. Glass can cause a lot of trouble; it can hide in places where you would never imagine it to be (Fig. 55), only to let its presence be known days or weeks later by a lump, infection or persistent pain. Most glass will show up on a soft tissue film if a radiograph is taken. A very thorough examination of all the crevices of a wound is essential if glass is the cause. This is especially important when a patient's face has been damaged by windscreen glass. The entry wound can be minute and look trivial, but glass can be buried deep inside cushioned by minute haematomas so that it cannot be felt easily. Any wound which has been caused by glass and subse-

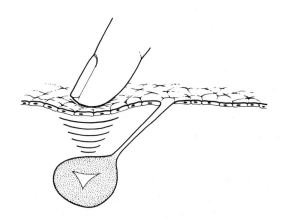

Fig. 55. *How glass fragments can 'hide' in a small haematoma.*

quently becomes infected should make you think of the possibility of a foreign body.

Seepage from wounds. Following suture, minor seepage from wounds can easily be controlled by pressure over the wound and elevation of a limb. Forehead and scalp wounds in particular, with their good blood supply, often require a few minutes direct pressure or even a pressure bandage for 12 hours to control the bleeding. Wounds of the face should not require any dressing at all. If the wound is covered it tends to remain soggy and can produce painful problems during removal of dressings. Advise the patient to have a clean cotton pillowcase that evening.

The eyebrow. If there is a wound in or near the eyebrow, do not shave the hair. Your patient will remain 'bald' and unsightly for a very long time and will not thank you for it if he wants to go to a dance or the like.

The lip. Suture of the lip has to be particularly accurate if a cut at the junction of the lip and ordinary skin ocurs, otherwise an unsightly mess will result. With all lacerations to the chin or round the lips, examine the inside of the mouth. A wound of the inside will often have been caused by the teeth and if deep will require suture. Later infection of the lip wound is common. To help avoid this ask the patient to dry the wound after all meals or drinks.

The tongue. Lacerations to the tongue hardly ever require suture. It should be explained to the patient that it will readily heal up without suture and advice should be given about a soft diet for the first few days. The doctor may prescribe antibiotics and ask the patient to have mouthwashes.

Dressings. All wounds, whether sutured or closed with Steristrips, should have a non-stick dressing, where needed, to help the nurse who has to take the dressing off. It is indefensible for a child to be crying when having an ordinary adherent dressing removed. One final point, just because a dressing is non-stick does not mean that it will come off 'like a dream'. Always edge it off carefully and have forceps ready to ease off any adherent sutures. If the dressing still sticks soak it in normal saline or an antiseptic solution until it peels off easily.

I have found the new conforming surgical tapes such as 'Hypafix' to be extremely useful for holding dressings in place in awkward places. It comes in several sizes. In many instances it can replace 'Netalast'.

Grazes. Although not serious, grazes are painful; your patient will appreciate any gentleness which can be afforded. The essential thing is to remove the dirt. When young lads come off motor bikes, grazing can be extensive and the dressing can take anything up to an hour to complete efficiently. Cleaning is best done with a mixture of Savlon and hydrogen peroxide. Buried gravel can be picked out with splinter forceps. As a dressing I prefer some form of *tulle* such as Bactigras with Melolin or other non-stick dressing on top of it, then a pad and crêpe bandage.

Skin glue. A new product has recently been launched on the market. It is a tissue adhesive which could well have a very useful or interesting place in the treatment of wounds. I have no experience of its use at the moment but it could prove to have a place, after sufficient trials have been performed.

Suture removal

Just because a doctor has asked you to remove the sutures, does not necessarily mean that they are ready to come out. Wounds which have initially been contaminated often taken longer to heal than similar wounds on a ward. Added to this is the considerable factor of patient activity and interference. With this in mind, it is a far safer approach always to remove alternate sutures first to see if the wound holds together. If it does not hold, Steristrips can be applied between the remaining sutures to strengthen it. With delicate wounds of the face, where the sutures have to be removed early to prevent scarring, place Steristrips across the wound after the removal of each suture to prevent the tragedy of the wound opening up again. A No. 11 scalpel blade is far better for taking out these minute sutures. Always pull the suture out in the direction of the wound (Fig. 56).

Nerve and tendon damage

If nerve or tendon damage is suspected, check the sensations of the surrounding skin and distal parts. With a limb ensure that no

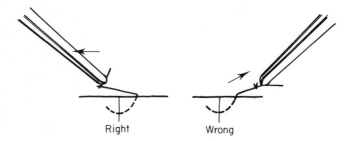

Fig. 56. *Removal of sutures. If the suture is removed towards the wound its edges are still held together. If pulled away from the wound, traction is applied to the edges and it may burst open.*

tendons have been damaged by asking the patient to put all the joints through a full range of movement. Repairing damage to an extensor tendon in the hand can be a comparatively simple procedure; with the flexor tendons a completely different picture appears and repair can be a long and difficult operation involving grafting. Unless the injury is very 'clean', the definitive operation will be delayed many weeks until tissue reaction has settled down.

Foreign bodies

On the subject of foreign bodies, glass has already been mentioned and I will not dwell on it any longer. There are, however, many other types of foreign body which commonly occur and these deserve special mention.

Wood splinters sometimes cause trouble in the skin of the fingers and palm of the hand. Even if you cannot see or feel them, please believe your patient. In many cases which I have seen, patients have been proved to be right time after time when the doctor doubted them. A hidden splinter is often the site of a recurrent or continual infection. If the end of the splinter cannot be held with forceps, an injection of lignocaine will be given into a bloodless field so that an incision can be made to find the splinter. Never underestimate the difficulty which is sometimes found in locating a foreign body. It can bring the most able surgeon to his knees.

Wood splinters beneath the nail are very common; once again, they have to be removed otherwise infection will supervene. The

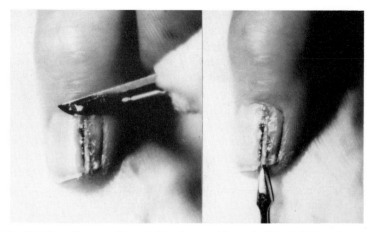

Fig. 57. *The nail over a splinter is shaved away with a scalpel blade. Splinter forceps are then used to grasp the end.*

majority of patients have already 'had a go' at removing the splinter and, of course, will have broken the end off. The easiest and surest method is to shave down the overlying nail using a scalpel blade (No. 15). This will take many minutes to do, but is practically painless for the patient until you get down to near where the splinter is (Fig. 57). Once all the nail over the splinter is removed, the end can be easily grasped with splinter forceps.

About three-quarters of puncture wounds to the foot, which are usually caused by nails, leave some dirt inside. Bearing this in mind, it is always worth while looking inside with splinter forceps and cleaning the minute wound properly. It is negligent simply to wipe over the surface of the skin with a swab.

WOUNDS OF THE CHEST OR ABDOMEN

Never underestimate a chest or abdominal wound. A seemingly small graze or bruise can overlie severe internal damage.

Stab wounds can be rapidly fatal, so all patients must be examined thoroughly and radiographs taken. It is well worth while speaking at some length with the patient to find out exactly how the stabbing occurred. By doing this you can gain an impression of the size of blade, direction of stab and depth of the wound. In all but the most trivial wounds an intravenous infusion will be required: not because the patient requires any volume replacement, but just to keep the vein open in case of deterioration. Give the patient nothing by mouth until it is decided what is to happen. Keep the patient on frequent charting of pulse and blood pressure so that deterioration can be noticed quickly.

A large abdominal wound with coils of intestine presenting (burst abdomen) is not such a terrible injury as it first appears. The patient should be positioned so that he is either lying flat with the knees bent up a little or sitting up with the knees bent, depending on which position gives most comfort. Cover the exposed intestine with sterile gamgee soaked in normal saline. Reassurance is high on the list of priorities, along with other general resuscitative measures.

PREVENTION OF TETANUS

The first and surest way of preventing tetanus is thorough cleaning and debriding of the wound; nothing can take its place. Secondly the public at large should be immunized so that they are always protected. A large proportion of tetanus cases are caused by comparatively trivial wounds. The patient may not even seek medical advice.

For complete active immunization a full course of three injections of absorbed tetanus vaccine is given: the initial dose is 0.5 ml; a booster dose of 0.5 ml is given 6 to 12 weeks later and a final booster dose of 0.5 ml 6 to 12 months later. Immunity will not have reached a satisfactory level until after the second injection. After a course of three injections, immunity will be satisfactory for five years, but this depends to some extent on the severity of the injury. For example, a tiny clean scratch will not require further injection, whereas a large wound with dead and devitalized tissue will.

If immediate, passive protection against tetanus is required, human tetanus immunoglobulin can be given, 250 i.u. is an average dose. If given with tetanus vaccine it must be injected into a different site with a different syringe and needle.

A long-acting penicillin is also sometimes given as a second line of defence against tetanus, for example, benzathine or Triplopen intramuscularly. If you give penicillin to anyone on the unit, always check first to see if they are allergic. Even though the doctor will already have asked, an extra 'safety net' is always of use.

Reactions to the immunoglobulin and vaccine are not very common. Mostly, they consist of local redness, swelling and pain at the injection site occurring a day or days later; this will pass off of its own accord.

PREVENTION OF RABIES

Thanks to our island state and strict quarantine laws, if a patient receives an animal bite in this country it is not necessary to give him rabies vaccine.

However, it is sometimes required for patients bitten, scratched or licked while on holiday abroad. If you are in doubt, your regional centre for infectious illnesses should be contacted. Advice can be sought from them 24 hours a day.

Note that it is not only dogs which may pass on the disease; cats, donkeys, foxes, rodents and many more can all pass on the disease. The infecting animal may appear well at the time of the bite or scratch. Treatment of patients following a suspected rabies contact consists of a course of six injections given at specified intervals.

THE EMBEDDED FISH HOOK

Every fishing season brings its trail of young boys and veteran fishermen who have a hook embedded in their skin. The hook is barbed (Fig. 58) so that it cannot simply be pulled out. First ask the patient either to draw or to describe what the hook looks like, as some have several barbs. The finger should be anaesthetized using either local anaesthesia or ethyl chloride spray. Guided by the drawing of the hook, push it so that the point will carry on through the skin and pierce the surface. After that either cut off the barb with wire cutters and withdraw the hook through its entry wound or cut off the eye and pull it out of the exit wound. On rare occasions, if the metal breaks off inside, an incision will have to be made. If ethyl chloride is being used, wait for the skin to 'thaw' a little, otherwise it will be like pushing through solid ice. Extreme cold also tends to make the hook brittle.

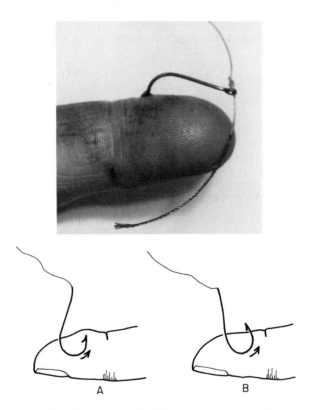

Fig. 58. *An embedded fish hook and its removal.*

THE DISAPPEARING BUTTERFLY

Many women, some men and surprisingly some very young girls have their ears pierced so that ear-rings can be worn. After the ear is pierced, the hole is often kept open with little gold studs held in place by a gold spring which looks a little like a butterfly. It is not unusual for this butterfly to retract inside the pinna of the ear, making it impossible for the patient to remove it. Matters are then made worse by infection. Removal is fairly simple, requiring no anaesthetic at all (Fig. 59). The rounded end of the gold stud is held firmly, either with the fingernails or with fine artery forceps. The stud is pushed in further while at the same time the skin on the other side is retracted. This will show at least part of the butterfly.

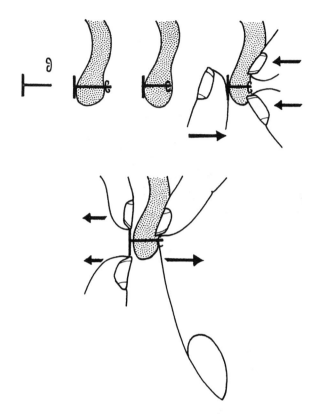

Fig. 59. *Removal of a 'butterfly' ear-ring.*

The loops of the butterfly are opened with fine curved mosquito forceps and can be pulled out of the pinna. Cutting is never required and local anaesthetic will cause more pain than the removal, although ethyl chloride spray may sometimes prove to be ideal.

HIGH PRESSURE INJURIES

In industry, water, oil and grease are frequently used under very high pressure for cleaning and lubricating. If, by accident, the jet hits the body, very serious damage can be done. The site of injury is usually the hand or arm. Frequently, the entry wound is small, but the substance can be forced unsuspected through the tissues, causing widespread damage. An inflammation of the tissues and damage to the blood supply will soon ensue and urgent decompression may be required to spare the circulation to the digits.

STINGS AND BITES

As you well know, an ordinary bee or wasp sting causes only moderate local reaction and discomfort. If you look closely at the site of a bee sting, the 'sting' may be seen and should be carefully removed intact. In all probability all that will then be required is something such as an antihistamine cream applied locally, after the area has been cleaned. Insect bites are very common during the summer months and are found most often on the lower legs following a walk in the garden or in grass. The patient often does not remember being bitten and just comes complaining of a very painful local reaction. The lesion often becomes very severe requiring antibiotics and/or antihistamines. Blisters which appear on the leg will require dressing and the leg, often very swollen, will need firm bandaging.

Snake bites

In the UK snake bites are fairly uncommon, although this obviously depends on the site of your department. The adder is the only poisonous snake which is native to the British Isles. The most common snake to be found is the grass snake, the bite of which is harmless except for the local reaction which can occur with any bite. If a patient comes complaining of a snake bite, recognition of the species involved is of obvious importance. The patient should be asked to describe the snake in detail and should be shown pictures if possible. The snake, however, is often not seen. The site of the bite, usually the ankle or hand, should be examined carefully. The bite will usually consist of two puncture marks, which may be difficult to see at first. The patient should be laid on a trolley, spoken to very reassuringly, and the temperature, pulse, respiration and blood pressure taken. The site of the bite will require cleaning and anti-tetanus toxoid should be given (this alone will help the patient mentally a great deal). If the snake was known to be a grass snake the patient can be allowed home. If the snake could not be identified, observation of the patient will be necessary, at least overnight. Even if the bite was known to have been made by an adder, a policy of 'wait and see' should be adopted because in many instances only mild local and/or constitutional symptoms will be noted, whereas treatment can have its own side-effects.

Throughout the country, each region has special hospitals which have been designated for storing snake venom. Advice should be sought from them about the patient's further care.

A STICKY PROBLEM

Over recent years a new type of glue, 'super glue' or 'Loctite', has been available which will bond human skin, among other things, in a matter of seconds. If a patient arrives with this problem, the manufacturers suggest soaking the part in warm soapy water and using a peeling, shearing force to separate the surfaces rather than to pull them apart. The blunt end of an instrument such as a McDonald's dissector may be useful to prise the edges apart without damaging the skin. Surgery should never be required.

On one occasion I have seen the glue cause a blister to rise on the skin. When the clothing was removed the upper layer of skin came away with it. Treatment was as for a burn blister.

The funniest occasion I can remember (for me, not the patient) was when a bus driver walked in through the doors holding on to his bus steering wheel, his hand firmly attached at the palm!

PARAPHIMOSIS

Paraphimosis is a condition which occurs mostly in teenagers. It is caused by a tight foreskin being left retracted and is usually discovered the next morning, following the previous night's sexual activities.

Conservative treatment is painful, but successful in the majority of instances. Depending on the severity of the condition one or a combination of the following can be attempted:

- Traction plus manipulation of the foreskin over the glans
- Hyaluronidase injections locally
- Packing ice round the penis followed by traction

BLAST INJURIES

Thankfully, blast injuries are not a major problem in the majority of accident and emergency departments, but the potential of a bomb incident hangs over us all. Injuries from a given form of road traffic accident can be predictable to some extent. However, the same cannot be said of blast injuries. Action must follow the same routine as mentioned in Chapters 2 and 3, that is, energetic resuscitation followed by the usual rules of reception. It would, however, be sensible to go just a little into the background of what happens in a blast and especially its effects on the body. Following an explosion, the blast wave can be thought of as being like a gust of wind travelling at an unbelievably fast speed and lessening in force the further you are from it. It can even flow round obstructions and be reflected from one surface to another.

The effect of this blast on a victim is like a blow to the whole of the body. The force of this blow carries on through the various tissues causing damage on the way, especially to organs which are filled with gas. Added to this is the fact that the body is usually thrown through the air by the blast landing against windows, walls or debris causing more injuries. Obviously the closer a person is to the blast the worse will be the effects. This will vary from complete disintegration of the body on top of the explosion, through to limbs being torn off a short distance away and perhaps just the occasional laceration and ear trouble at a distance (Fig. 60).

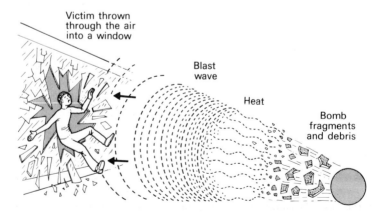

Fig. 60. *The effects of a bomb blast.*

Added to the effects mentioned so far, we must add that bomb fragments and debris will be thrown against our victim. The bomb fragments will be of irregular shape and travelling at a high velocity like rifle bullets. They will therefore cause much damage to the body tissues.

Our bomb blast patients, therefore, can have a mixture of injuries with different causative mechanisms:

- Blast $\rightarrow$ deafness; lung damage; amputations
- Heat $\rightarrow$ burns of varying severity
- Bomb fragments $\rightarrow$ high-velocity missile wounds
- Debris hitting patient $\rightarrow$ multiple wounds; fractures
- Body hitting a window, wall, etc. $\rightarrow$ multiple wounds; fractures

GUNSHOT WOUNDS

Shootings, although not an everyday occurrence in Great Britain, are rapidly increasing in number. Because of this, I wish to spend just a little time stressing the important points in the care of these injuries.

The type of damage caused by gunshot wounds will depend on the type of weapon used. This can be of a high or low velocity. Low-velocity missiles, for instance from hand guns, cause *comparatively* little damage. Most damage is made directly by the passage of the missile itself through the tissues (Fig. 61). Injuries caused by high-velocity weapons, for instance rifles, can be far more extensive. The reason for this is two-fold. Firstly, a shock wave precedes the passage of the missile through the tissues by a fraction of a second. This causes damage at a distance from the tract. Parts of the body which are more solid tend to be the worst affected, i.e. muscle, liver, spleen. Secondly, something called temporary cavitation occurs, which follows the passage of the missile by a fraction of a second causing tremendous damage. The tissues on either side of the missile are moved forwards and outwards producing a momentary cavity, sometimes 30 to 40 times the diameter of the missile (Fig. 62), thereby pulping soft tissue in the area or shattering a bone. As the cavity occurs it creates a suction. Air contaminated with the debris is sucked into the missile tract. The sheer power of a high-velocity missile can be hard for us to appreciate because it is not something which we can see

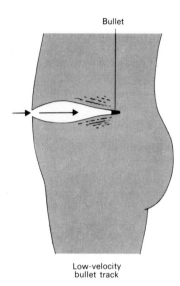

Fig. 61. *The damage caused by a low-velocity missile.*

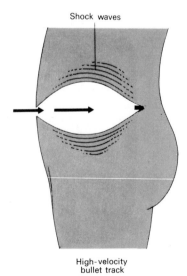

Fig. 62. *The damage caused by a high-velocity missile.*

directly. A good example of this is that large blood vessels, because they are somewhat elastic, can be pushed aside and appear undamaged, however, the inner lining can be damaged leading to a thrombosis hours later.

The final damage of the missile injury cannot therefore be realized solely by the external appearance of the wound. We must also obtain a history of the incident to try to find which type of weapon may have been used and the possible direction of entry.

Surgical methods for such injuries differ widely from the standard repairs done in everyday trauma, but are far beyond the scope of this book. Suffice it to say that extensive exploration and debridement is often required, followed by loose packing; secondary suture will be required about five days later. This 'wartime' treatment saved the lives of so many of our soldiers in the Falklands' war. Resuscitation in the accident and emergency department may have to be very active if the patient is to survive and this must be followed by rapid transfer to theatre. In such circumstances speed is of the essence.

Airgun pellets

Here we have a completely different situation. The people injured are usually children, which is I suppose a reflection of the far too easy availability of such weapons. The pellets usually lie fairly superficially and produce little local damage. The main danger seems to be injury to the eyes. However beware, at close range they can penetrate a considerable distance and are potentially lethal.

Be alert to a new type of airgun pellet on the market, part of which is made of plastic and therefore does not show up on x-rays.

FURTHER READING

Cain, D. & Weeks, R.F. (1983) A new danger associated with airgun pellets. *British Medical Journal*, 286.
Conolly, W. & Kilgore, E. (1979) *Hand injuries and infections*, 1st edn. London: Edward Arnold.
Owen Smith, M.S. (1981) *High-velocity missile wounds*. London: Edward Arnold.

7   Burns and scalds

Severe pain, weeks of discomfort, life-long mental torment of disfigurement or even death can all await some of the unfortunate burn victims. However, even in the accident and emergency unit our care can ease the pain considerably, give hope to the worried relatives and make all the difference between life and death. The handling of a dressing on a lesser injury can likewise alter its eventual duration and outcome.

GENERAL CARE OF BURN PATIENTS

When you initially see the patient, the burns themselves have such a visual impact that it is difficult to consider damage elsewhere, but your priority is to pay attention to the patient's general condition.

Resuscitation

Resuscitation is the primary objective in severe burns. Momentarily forget about the skin and consider the immediate life-endangering conditions:

1. Does the patient have a pulse?
2. Is the patient breathing?
3. Is the patient's airway clear?
4. Is the patient's circulation satisfactory?

After a fire, more people die from the effects of the smoke than from burns. Smoke affects the lungs, first by irritating, then by suffocating and perhaps hours later by causing pulmonary oedema. Danger signs are as follows:

1. Soot and scorched hair inside the nostrils
2. Cough
3. A feeling of tightness in the chest
4. Wheezing
5. A burning sensation inside the chest
6. Stridor

7. Burns to the lips
8. A husky voice

If air is getting in but the patient has distressed respirations give oxygen with an MC or similar mask. Deteriorating or more severe cases may require intubation and intermittent positive-pressure ventilation (IPPV) at any moment because of swelling of the upper airway, increasing respiratory embarrassment due to circumferential burns or pulmonary oedema. If the patient has a previous bad chest, for example, chronic bronchitis, the position may be very precarious indeed, with the patient requiring urgent intensive therapy. Although there are doubtless circumstances when emergency tracheostomy is an essential life-saving procedure, its use in severe burns is not ideal. If the patient can be intubated initially, tracheostomy is far better performed in a day or so, when the condition is more stable. It can then be performed as an elective procedure by a surgeon who is used to the operation. Cutting through circumferential, deeply burnt areas of the chest wall (escharotomy) is sometimes also necessary to ease failing respirations.

Our next essential is to set up an intravenous infusion of human plasma protein fraction (HPPF). This will be required for most burns over 10 per cent in a child and 15 per cent in an adult.

One simple method of estimating the percentage of skin which has been burnt is Wallace's rule of nine (Fig. 63). This simple system divides the body roughly up into areas of 9 per cent (Table 4). It does not matter whether the burn is partial or full thickness, all burnt areas count except simple erythema.

Some difficulty may be encountered initially in finding an injection site because of the burns. If this occurs, a cut down through the burnt area will be required.

To find the rate that the infusion should run, make the following calculation:

$$\frac{\text{percentage of burns} \times \text{patient's weight (kg)}}{2}$$

= No. of ml in 4 hours

e.g.
$$\frac{50\% \text{ burns} \times 60 \text{ kg}}{2} = \frac{3000}{2} = 1500 \text{ ml every 4 hours}$$

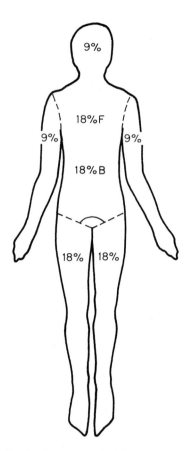

Fig. 63. *Wallace's rule of nine: a method for estimating the area of burns.*

At this stage do not think of the burns in isolation. If the patient has been involved in a road accident or explosion, for instance, consider the likely problems of head injury, limb fractures and rupture of abdominal viscera. Even if smoke has not been a problem at the scene, 'blast lung' can cause later chest complications which can be just as vicious.

Analgesia is required for the majority of patients. Morphine or pethidine is usual, either intramuscularly or intravenously.

Catheterization, although it may ultimately be necessary, is not an emergency procedure and can be done better when the patient

Table 4. *Wallace's rule of nine: division of the body into areas of 9 per cent.*

	%
Head	9
Each arm	9
Front of each leg	9
Back of each leg	9
Front of chest	9
Back of chest	9
Front of abdomen	9
Back of abdomen	9
Perineum	1

is settled on the ward, rather than unnecessarily blocking up the accident and emergency unit.

With severe or extensive burns, a lot will depend on local hospital policy as to whether or not they will be dressed on the accident and emergency unit. Certainly they will require careful assessement with drawings by a senior surgeon before they are finally 'wrapped up'. Also the accident and emergency senior nurse should ensure that the often long and complex dressing of such patients does not impinge on the space and staff available for reception of further major injuries.

The appearance of the burnt area

Many old classifications of the depth of a burn are still used to this day. This is to be discouraged. The universal classification is now as follows:

1. Partial thickness
2. Full thickness

It is not always as easy as it seems to tell exactly what is partial and what is full thickness. Sometimes several days waiting will be necessary until the definition is clear. Here are some general rules:

Erythema ⎫
Blistering ⎭   *Partial*   The patient can still feel pin pricks

Creamy white skin ⎫
Brown   *Deep*   The full thickness areas will be anaesthetic
Black   ⎭

The local care of the burn

There is a problem with lesser burns in that there may well be a wait before the doctor is able to see the patient. Apart from drugs there is but one effective way of immediately easing the pain of a burn patient. That is simply to immerse the part in cold water or place it under the tap. Alternatively some measure of relief will be gained by sterile moist dressings. A good temporary cover, easing some pain and also allowing the doctor to see the burnt surface is 'cling' kitchen film. The principles of dressings are:

1. The patient should be in a clean atmosphere, that is, in a clean dressing room or a theatre.
2. Clean up the surrounding skin if necessary. Often a whole limb will have to be placed in a bowl and washed to remove all the soot. Until this has been done it would be a waste of time attending to the burnt surface.
3. From now on, using full aseptic technique, clean the burnt surface, removing any damaged dirty blisters using scissors and forceps.
4. Incise any unbroken blisters and express the fluid (Fig. 64).
5. Apply a non-stick dressing, for example:
   (a) *Tulle* plus gauze
   (b) *Tulle* plus Melolin

On top of the initial dressing apply a substantial layer of gamgee, since there will be a large fluid loss through the burnt area during the first 48 hours. Finish off the dressing with a firm crêpe or cotton bandage. Ensure that the dressing gives a good overlap onto good skin and that the final bandages go even further. You would be surprised what some patients get up to when they leave the department; plenty of bandages improve the dressings' 'patient impregnability'! On no account have the bandage too loose; if this

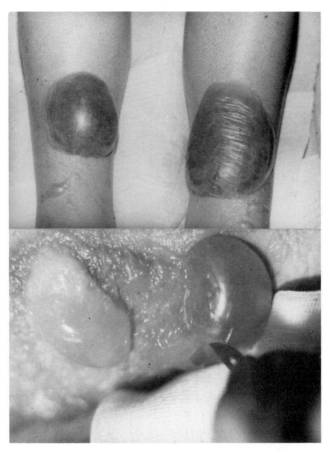

Fig. 64. *Intact blisters can be punctured with a scalpel blade and the fluid expressed. Leave the blistered skin in situ; it makes the area feel more comfortable for the patient and does not delay healing.*

occurs shearing forces will cause pain at the slightest movement. If the patient is to be allowed home warn of possible seepage so that he will not worry too much. If the burnt area is large advise the patient to drink plenty of fluids. Review the burnt area after two days to ensure that seepage is contained and that no more blistering has occurred. It is not necessary at this stage to remove the final layer of *tulle* next to the burnt skin; to do so can impede wound healing. Op-Site used instead of dressings shows promise in

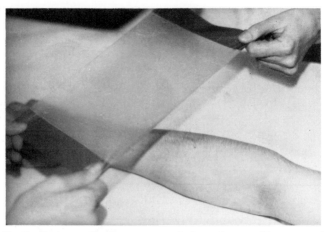

Fig. 65. *Op-Site in use. The film must cover the burned area and have an overlap of about 5 cm onto the surrounding skin.*

some cases (Fig. 65). With full-thickness or infected burns, creams are used (for instance silver sulphadiazine) to assist in the removal of slough. As the dressings progress, part of the slough is cut away as it loosens and more cream is applied.

Review of burn dressings

Brief mention is made here of the removal of burn dressings when the patient comes back to the clinic. This must always be done slowly, peeling away one layer of the dressing at a time with forceps. Often the dressing will have to be soaked off by dabbing over the hardened dressings with a Savlon swab. Callous pulling off is to be condemned. If the burn bleeds, you are being too rough and damaging the epithelium; it will therefore take longer to heal.

The ideal is for the dressing to be left alone for 10 to 14 days by which time healing should have occurred.

CHEMICAL BURNS

Chemical burns require special mention. The affected part must be flooded with water as soon as the patient enters the department. Although in most industrial cases first aid is excellent, it is always wise to 'double up' and do it again. Following this treatment the whole area can be covered with sterile gauze soaked in a 'buffer' solution. After this the treatment is the same as for any ordinary burn.

Hydrofluoric acid burns

Hydrofluoric acid is a really 'nasty' substance used in some industries. If splashed onto the skin it will continue to necrose tissue until bone is reached. After the usual washing, calcium gluconate jelly is applied to the skin. For a severe case calcium gluconate will have to be injected through a fine needle into and around the burnt area to ease the severe pain.

ELECTRICAL BURNS

With electrical burns we have two main problems. Firstly respiratory and cardiac arrhythmias or arrest; secondly, the burns can be very deep indeed. Even if the patient appears to be all right, he should have an ECG taken. Many patients feel extremely 'shaken up' for an hour or more after the incident.

SUNBURN

Sunburn is not common during an English summer, but with every hot spell we get a trail of unfortunates who have misjudged the sun. The effect is mainly that of erythema and blistering. Severe cases may have to be admitted, but this is uncommon and most are able to cope at home. Treatment is by smearing with a soothing cream. Advise the patient to keep as cool as possible when at home and to wear the minimum of clothing to prevent any rubbing. Patients with extensive sunburn often feel at the point of collapse, shivering, confused, drowsy and with a slightly raised or normal temperature. If this occurs keep the patient cool, give plenty of fluids and treat the burn as described above. If the burn is of moderate degree, the patient will be satisfactory at home; if it is severe, however, admission may be necessary.

THE SCALDED CHILD

The scalded child wrapped in blankets, crying and accompanied by worried, upset parents is a very common occurrence. A scald does hurt, no one will deny that, but as with adults the severity of the pain and the reaction to it can vary enormously. Some children will require drugs such as pethidine or trimeprazine immediately on admission. But also sit back for a moment and study the child and the parent. You will find that, if the mother is sensible and has been able to keep control of herself and is cuddling and comforting the child, the child will be quiet in a large proportion of cases or even sleeping. In this instance analgesia is not necessary. Even in the case of an upset crying child, with an explanation to the parents, the child can often be calmed considerably and therefore will not require analgesia.

When doing dressings on such children, prepare all your equipment first. For example, pour out the lotions, cut the *tulle* and open the bandages before the child is even brought into the room. This preparation will cut down the 'crying time' considerably. It only requires one screaming child to upset a waiting room full of children, quite apart from the distress to the child's parents. As with all dressings on babies and small children, bandage them very securely in position and strap the ends down with plenty of strapping to dissuade tiny fingers from prying. Wear gloves for the procedure for extra sensitivity. An experienced nurse should be with you together with the mother to hold the child steady; even babies can be tremendously strong and must be held firmly if the dressing is not to take a long time.

Before you begin, explain to the parents that the child will start crying as soon as you start the procedure but that it will hardly cause any pain. Most of the crying is due to the child being upset.

A final point, remember to be alert to the possibility of non-accidental injury.

THE HOUSE FIRE

One of the most upsetting times for a nurse on the accident and emergency unit is where a whole family has been in a house fire. One or several of the children may have been killed and the parents are both stunned and with varying degrees of burns themselves. What can you do to help the survivors? Despite feeling rather helpless at first, there are many ways in which you can help:

• Deal efficiently with their burns
• Be on the alert for signs of chest complications

- Keep the family together, even if they are on trolleys, so that they can see and talk to one another and gain some comfort
- Make them all a drink; find out if they want something to eat
- Perhaps most important of all, talk to them and be a good *listener*
- Help them get cleaned up and dressed temporarily in whatever clothes are available
- Get the help of others, for instance, relatives or priest, or the Social Services and the local housing department for temporary accommodation.

FURTHER READING

Cason, J.S. (1981) *Treatment of burns.* London: Chapman & Hall.
Wagner, M.M. (Ed.) (1981) *Care of the burn-injured patient.* London: Croom Helm.

8 An introduction to bone and joint injuries

The fields of accident and emergency and orthopaedics will forever intermix and a clear dividing line is impossible. In this chapter, the first of three on orthopaedic trauma, a general explanation of basic nursing points is given first. This is followed by sections on plaster of Paris technique, exercises, crutches, muscular injuries and radiography.

THE STATE OF THE LIMB

The most important item which a nurse must bear in mind when caring for any orthopaedic patient is to be sure that the state of the limb is satisfactory. By this I mean that she must check the following points personally.

1. That the *circulation* to the limb is intact
2. That *sensations* of the limb are normal
3. That *movements* of affected parts are normal
4. That there is no excessive *swelling*
5. That the *skin* is not being damaged
6. That whatever *splint*, plaster or bandage is on is in a good state and doing its job correctly
7. That there is no unaccountable *pain*

Never is this more important than in an accident and emergency department, where the patients are often critically ill, or in out-patients, who will not be seen again for a week or more.

Circulation of the limb

First look at the limb or the part of it which is not covered by splint or bandage. Skin with a good circulation tends to be mainly pink. If it is white or mottled, little or no blood is getting through. If it is blue or congested there may be obstruction of the venous return. To be sure, compare with the 'good' side. Remember that following fractures, blood often tracks down the limb to the fingers or toes making them bruised, and warn your patients about this.

Pressure on the finger or toenails can also be a useful guide. The normal nail bed is a good deep pink. If you press this, it should blanch. As your release the pressure it should return once again to the original colour fairly quickly. In the case of an ischaemic limb, if the nail bed is not white already, pressure will once again make it so, but the colour will either not return or return only slowly. If the opposite occurs, for example the colour returns quicker than normal, this indicates that there is some degree of venous obstruction.

Next, touch the skin; an ischaemic limb will be cold unless the injury has only just occurred. Once again compare this with the 'good' side. Extra warmth is a pointer to infection being the cause of the trouble.

Pulses should be your final confirmation of the state of the circulation. Compare both sides of the body, especially if you have difficulty in finding one on the injured limb. Even with a plaster cast on, if the circulation to the limb is in doubt, a pulse can easily be felt for by making a small cut or window in the plaster over the usual site. A very useful pulse called the dorsalis pedis is found on the dorsum of the foot (Fig. 66). The radial pulse should be very familiar to you all and its neighbour, the ulnar, is not too hard to find.

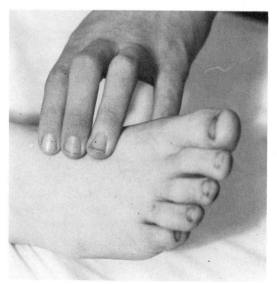

Fig. 66. *Taking the dorsalis pedis pulse.*

Sensations to the limb

Except in some instances at the roadside, when the patient's limb is momentarily 'numbed', the sensations of a limb following a fracture should be as normal as yours or mine. Touch the limb distal to the fracture or dislocation to ensure that the patient can feel you. Do this in several places so that you do not miss a small yet important area of trouble. Next, ask the patient if there are any 'pins and needles', 'tingling' or numbness anywhere (paraesthesia). If present, this indicates pressure somewhere on the nerve supplying the part. Fig. 67 shows the nerve distribution to the skin of the hand.

Movements of the limb

By movements, I do not mean that you are to move the fractured limb, merely, see if the patient can move, for instance, the fingers

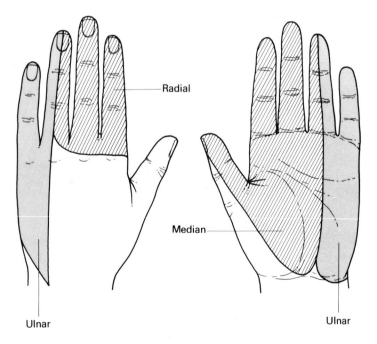

Fig. 67. *The nerve distribution to the skin of the hand.*

and toes distal to the injury. With the upper limb making a fist, straightening out the fingers and thumb and then spreading the fingers out and putting them together will test the action of the median, radial and ulnar nerves, respectively. With the foot, your patient should be able to bend and straighten the toes.

Swelling of a limb

Of all the possibilities remember first that swelling may have been there for some time and compare it with the other leg. Note also whether it is a collection of blood in the tissues, oedema, an effusion into a joint or associated with infection.

The most common of all 'orthopaedic swellings' is oedema caused by whatever splint, bandage or plaster the patient is wearing being too tight. If you apply any constricting force round a limb, even if it is spread out like a bandage, it will squeeze the veins and lymphatics causing back-pressure and therefore oedema in the tissues distal to it. Add to this a fracture or ruptured muscles, both with progressive bleeding, and you have a precarious position in which swelling occurs easily. Swelling is dangerous because, if severe, it can stop the arterial supply to the limb. Also, while it is present it will hinder the patient from regaining a full range of joint movement. A final thought for you on this subject: some traumatic orthopaedic conditions can cause an unsuspected deep vein thrombosis.

Skin

Always have in mind what the skin is like underneath the bandage. Look at the edges of splints or plasters for red skin where they may be digging in. Is there any increased warmth, any discharge or any pain which might indicate a plaster sore? Is there abnormal itching, indicating that the patient is allergic to some of the material used? Is the safety-pin stuck through the skin? It does happen!

Plaster

Make sure that the bandage, splint or plaster extends to the correct level, as shown later, and is firmly applied. With a plaster of Paris cast look for cracks, rough edges or soggy or soft areas.

Pain

With most orthopaedic injuries, even if expertly reduced and immobilized, some pain is to be expected. This must be explained to your patient. You will find that your patients are willing to put up with a far higher level of pain and discomfort as long as they know that it is to be expected for a short while. The next point is *never to treat pain with analgesics until you have found out its cause.* If you do not obey this rule, one day you will make a terrible mistake. Once the cause has been found, try to alleviate it first with adjustments to the patient's position or the splint, and resort to analgesics only if all else fails.

RADIOGRAPHY

On an accident and emergency unit radiographs are not the sole concern of the doctor. For the nurse to apply the various treatments personally or to assist the doctor intelligently with a reduction, she must see and study them and know what to look for. Many a busy casualty officer has been grateful for the additional scrutiny of a worried sister. Before adequate interpretation can be achieved, revision in depth of the anatomy of bones must be done, then followed up by the study of as many radiographs as you can possibly lay your hands on. It is only by this study and knowing what the normal is like that radiographs will ever be of any use to you.

How to study a film. Although it seems terribly obvious, do first check that the films are of the correct patient; mistakes are so easily made and can cause a lot of trouble. Next, ensure that the films are dated correctly and are of the correct side of the body. Always ensure that two radiographs of a patient are available, taken at right angles to one another. Look at the quality of the film. Is it too light or too dark and not showing up the detail of the bones clearly enough? Has it been taken at exactly the correct plane or at a slight angle, making interpretation difficult? Follow the outline of all the bones shown on the film looking for a break or step in the cortex even in places where the patient has no pain. If you come across a fracture, do not stop; carry on looking at the outline of all the other bones. When this is done then look at the inside of the bones for a line which could be a fracture. It can be helpful and stimulating for both parties if you discuss with the casualty officer anything unusual which you see. Just because there is no fracture shown on the radiograph, does not mean that there is no fracture there. The radiograph never lies, but often it does not tell you the whole truth! If the doctor is concerned about the injury, views from different angles or tomograms may have to be taken before a diagnosis can be made with certainty.

PLASTER OF PARIS TECHNIQUE

Before attempting to run you must learn to walk; before attempting to apply a plaster you must be fully competent at applying ordinary bandages. Here, I am giving you the basic principles so that you can make a reasonable attempt at common casts, that is, below the knee and short arm casts. These are the commonest and are done almost every day in an accident and emergency unit. The methods and materials may vary slightly in your own unit but the principles are the same. Never apply one on a patient until you have practised beforehand on one of your friends.

Helpers. No matter how skilled the nurse who applies the plaster, all the work will be to no avail if she cannot rely on someone knowledgeable to hold the limb in the correct position. This should be the task of your most senior assistant because it is of such importance. It is worse than useless having a plaster which looks superb but holds the limb in the incorrect position; this will encourage people to 'make do' and leave it in the poor position.

It is a sad but vital fact in these litigation-minded days that if you are a male nurse, a chaperon in the form of a relative or another nurse is essential for your own protection. This is especially true in an accident and emergency unit where you seldom get to know your patient thoroughly or personally.

Explanation. Especially to children, but also to many adults, the application of a plaster is enshrouded in mystery. Where there is mystery, there is fear and this must be allayed. Most will understand if you relate it to the application of an ordinary bandage.

If the application is going to be painful at times and the patient is a child, never lie by saying it will not hurt. Play down the pain by all

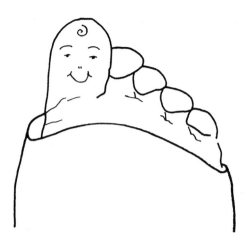

Fig. 68. *Children in the accident and emergency unit require special care.*

means, but the patient's cooperation, which is very useful to you, depends on trust. I remember that in my childhood, part of the fear of going to the dentist was the horrifying sight of the clinical-looking room and its grotesque machinery. The plaster room with its tools and machinery must add to the apprehension of small children. How much more pleasant it would be, even in a general hospital, if the walls were decorated with posters, toys were available in every room and nurses played with the children (Fig. 68).

Equipment. The room requires a sturdy table which will tilt for a general anaesthetic. Some form of plaster trolley is ideal, although not essential. A good supply of old newspapers and plenty of plastic sheeting for the inevitable spillages are also vital. You must wear a substantial apron which practically touches the floor and sturdy rubber boots. Even with all this protection it is amazing how the plaster still finds your clothing. If the odd spot does land on your clothes, wait for it to dry before you attack it. When dry, pick it off with the edge of a knife blade and then use a firm brush for what is left.

The basic instruments required for the above simple plaster work are:

Shears, in several sizes and designs
Bandage scissors
Spreaders
Electric plaster saw

Collect whatever plaster bandages you will require and tear open the packets. Do not take them out of the papers; if they are not used they can then be re-wrapped and saved for another time. Leaving the bandages opened but in the packets also helps to stop the odd splash of water ruining them. An example of the number of rolls required for an adult is shown in Table 5. Exact numbers vary from nurse to nurse. The type of patient also has a bearing on the number required; for example, a teenager who is going to be very active will require a thicker cast than an old lady. Lastly, the

Table 5. *Number and type of bandages used for various plasters.*

Type of plaster	Type of bandage		
	Width		No. required
	(cm)	(in)	
Long leg	15	6	6
	20	8	6
Below knee	15	6	6
Cylinder	20	8	7
Short arm	7.5	3	1
	10	4	3
Long arm	7.5	3	1
	10	4	6
Scaphoid	5	2	1
	7.5	3	1
	10	4	3
Colles' slab	15	6	1

type of fracture plays a part. A trivial one may be allowed weight-bearing and will therefore require a heavier plaster than someone who will continually be in bed or on crutches.

The bucket or bowl of water can vary in temperature depending on how fast you want the plaster to set. With cold water the plaster sets slowly; with warm water it sets quickly. If you are inexperienced start with the water fairly cold so that you will have time to put the bandage on before hardening starts. As you improve, increase the temperature until it is warm. Never have the water hot; the heat of this plus the heat of the chemical change which takes place in the plaster can be enough to cause a burn.

Preparation of the patient. The patient will not thank you if you do not protect his clothing adequately. So if a leg plaster is being applied, trousers will in most cases have to be removed. Plaster washes off underclothes easily, so they can be left on. In no circumstances apply a long leg plaster with trousers, even old ones, just rolled up: you will not be able to apply it high enough up the thigh. It is, however, acceptable to do a below-knee plaster with the trousers just rolled up, *if* the patient has on wide, flared, old ones which he is not concerned about. In either case, the 'good' leg will have to be protected by plastic sheeting, as will the upper part of the body. A rest is then placed behind the knee to give support while the foot is held by your assistant (Fig. 69).

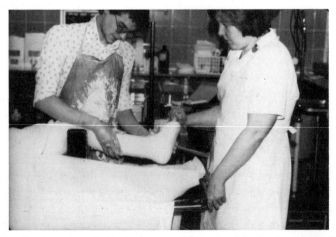

Fig. 69. *An assistant holds the foot at a right angle while the plaster is applied.*

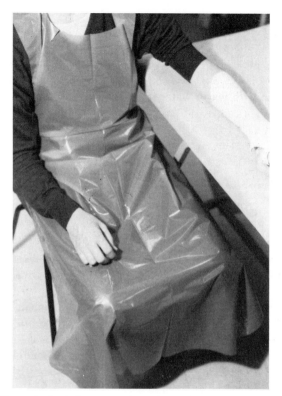

Fig. 70. *The patient's clothing must always be well protected while the plaster is being applied.*

With simple arm fractures, for example, an undisplaced Colles' or a scaphoid fracture, the patient will be all right sitting at the side of the table. The patient's clothing will have to be protected and he will have to keep his feet well tucked in under the chair so that no splashes reach the shoes (Fig. 70).

Technique. A layer of stockinette and/or orthopaedic wool is the first stage. This must be wrapped round the limb smoothly without wrinkles. If wrinkles and ridges are made in the wool the plaster will later mould to this shape, causing rigid uneven sections on the inner layer of the plaster. A simple method keeping the foot at right

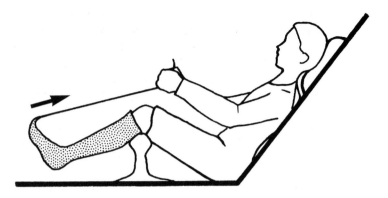

Fig. 71. *With minor injuries the foot can be kept at right angles using tube-gauze.*

angles while plastering and using tube-gauze is shown in Fig. 71 but this can only be employed, of course, in comparatively painless injuries.

Unravel a few centimetres of the end and immerse the bandage, resting it in the hand. Wait a few moments for most of the bubbles to escape, then lift it out and squeeze out excess water with both hands. Do not have it too dry or too wet; there should be just the occasional drip. To make sure that no drops of water drip over the dry bandages, position the bandages, water and patient so that they are all in a line.

Apply the bandage firmly against the orthopaedic wool with the right hand while the other smoothes the previous turn. This action is essential to smooth out the inside of the plaster, moulding it to the contours of the limb. Another effect it has is to compress the bandage layers together, giving the whole plaster of Paris far greater strength.

As a general rule, start bandaging at the fingers or toes and work upwards as you would normally, covering a portion of the previous turn. Try to let the bandage 'run' as best you can, but there are bound to be places where it will not apply smoothly. When this occurs, make small tucks and smooth them in as well. Do not try to keep to any regular pattern with the bandage, but apply it in a uniform thickness throughout the whole limb. If the plaster is thicker in one place than in another it will tend to crack at the junction of the two thicknesses.

Over joints such as the elbow, never just wrap the bandage round; this will result in a very thick portion on the inner aspect of the joints and not enough on the outside (Fig. 72). A far better result is obtained if you zig-zag the bandage over the outer surface, thereby preventing bunching up on the inside. Similarly zig-zagging can be of use in the hand, producing a strong bar between the thumb and index finger, yet not adding to the weight too much.

Any moulding and smoothing must be done with the flat of the hand. Using individual fingers may cause 'dints' which cannot be removed. Once these have dried they will cause continuous localized pressure and the common result is a sore.

With long leg and long arm plasters you will find it easier if the distal part of the plaster is completed first. The distal part can then be held more easily until all the plaster is done. The edges are made by turning back the stockinette and/or orthopaedic wool and plastering up to it. If this is done skilfully there should be no need for final trimming.

Never have the limb held in a particular position, plaster over it and then alter that position. The plaster will buckle on the inside

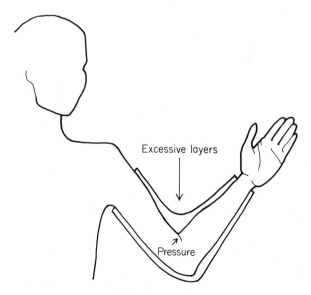

Fig. 72. *Simply wrapping a bandage round the elbow will cause excessive layers to build up on the inside and constrict the joint. Zig-zagging is better.*

causing a ridge, which will cause localized pressure in the hours ahead and give your patient at best severe discomfort.

If a walking plaster is applied, weight must not be applied to it for 48 hours, by which time the cast will have dried completely. To prevent patients being too adventurous, I only strengthen the sole with a slab when I initially apply the cast. Then when the patient comes for a check the next day, the heel is applied.

Aftercare. When completed, rest the cast throughout its length on something soft. Although the plaster seems hard, it can still be easily dented.

Explain the 'Dos and Don'ts' about plaster care to the patient. These are mainly:

1. If the patient has the slightest worry about it, he should phone or call in at any time
2. Support it on a soft surface
3. Do not get it wet
4. Keep it elevated
5. Exercise the fingers, toes and other joints
6. Expect some pain at the fracture site, especially in the first 24 hours
7. Tell the patient how and when to take analgesics
8. Tell the patient to observe the colour, temperature and sensation of the limb and what to do about what is found
9. Tell the patient the date of the next appointment
10. Do not heat the plaster to dry it out
11. Do not poke items down the plaster

Always ask the patient to return for a plaster check within the next 24 hours; it is surprising how many faults this will show up. One final point of aftercare: a very common mistake that patients with leg casts make, is to rest the heel on the floor; warn them of this, otherwise the plaster will soon require strengthening (Fig. 73).

Plaster removal

A plaster cast can either just be removed or be carefully split into two halves (bivalving).

Plaster shears are the main tool in our armoury. To work efficiently they have to be used with great care, the bottom handle

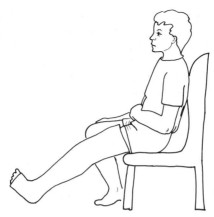

Fig. 73. *Resting the heel on the floor is a quick way to ruin a plaster.*

kept level with the plaster surface and only the top handle moving up and down. With some tight plasters, even if this rule is obeyed, it is hard not to injure the patient. To avoid injury always move the point forwards carefully and ask your patients if it is digging in before closing the jaws. I always try to imagine that it is my skin under there! I will never forget the time I had to remove a very tight plaster—it took me an hour so as not to hurt the patient. The cuts for removal and bivalving of a leg cast are done along the same lines (Fig. 74); with the arm, however, you can just cut up the front to remove it (Fig. 74) and for bivalving make two cuts. Take the greatest care at the inner fold of the elbow. After cutting, the edges will have to be separated with a spreader so that the underlying wool can be cut. The orthopaedic wool is then cut along the same line as the plaster. Bandage scissors and a lot of patience will be required for this because it can sometimes take longer than cutting the plaster.

Electric plaster saw. A saw operated electrically is a potentially dangerous tool and must be used with great care. It is very noisy, it vibrates and the sight of it is enough to send all but the brave running. With children its use should be reserved for large heavy plasters. It is important to understand the following points when using the plaster saw:

1. Have dry hands and keep away from oxygen
2. The blade does not rotate, it only oscillates (Fig. 75)

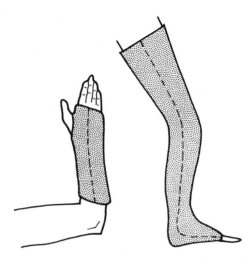

Fig. 74. *Cutting lines for the removal of a plaster. The leg plaster will have to be cut up both sides.*

3. If the saw is held in one place for more than a few seconds, heat will be produced and the patient may be burned
4. The saw vibrates and that is uncomfortable for the patient
5. It will only cut through hard surfaces, *not* the padding under the plaster of Paris
6. If you run the saw along the skin it will cut it; it you press down momentarily it will not

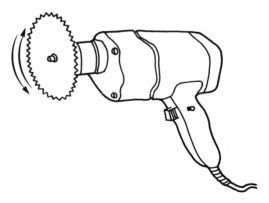

Fig. 75. *A plaster saw. Reassure your patient that the blade does not rotate.*

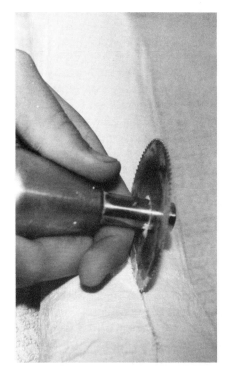

Fig. 76. *The correct way to hold a plaster saw.*

The saw is held in the right hand with the shaft resting on the operator's left fingers. This position gives you extra sensitivity (Fig. 76). To cut the plaster you press downwards. When it is cut through, the fingers of your left hand will feel it 'give'. Continue this up-and-down movement until the whole length of the plaster except the end by the skin has been done, then finish off with the shears.

Cast bracing. This is a method of immobilizing fractures while allowing movement of nearby joints. Many fractures can now be treated in this way and many centres are experimenting with this method of care. However, in most instances, this type of treatment does not come under the realm of accident and emergency care but is done days or weeks later in the treatment.

EXERCISES

I do not want to call this section 'physiotherapy' because that gives many nurses the impression that it is something that someone else does once a week. With orthopaedic trauma, however, it is something in which both you and your patient have to be very much involved. It is your job to teach your patient any exercises required to get the limbs strong again, it is also your task to check that he is continuing to do them and is progressing.

Arm exercises. A common example here is an old lady with a Colles' fracture. If just left alone the patient will leave the plastered arm in a sling because it hurts. The fingers will swell, muscles will weaken, shoulders stiffen. By the time the cast comes off the fracture will be healed but the arm will be useless.

What should happen is that the patient is taught exercises from the beginning. For the first day while the arm is still in a sling, the patient is shown how to make a fist actively, straighten the fingers and thumb right out, spread the fingers apart and put them together again. This will keep the muscles of the forearm in shape and help to 'pump' away oedema fluid and ease joint stiffness. Several times a day the arm is removed from the sling so that the patient can move the elbow and shoulder, which also helps to prevent stiffening. After 24 hours, when the sling is removed, the patient is encouraged to move the arm about, but not to have it hanging down. Coax the patient to use it for writing, holding *light* objects and dressing. If all the above is done, by the time the fracture is healed the patient will have a useful limb and will be well on the way to independence.

Leg exercises. As with the arm, it is also important to exercise an injured leg. It gives the patient a feeling of actively helping in the treatment so that he will soon be 'up and about' again. I will describe quadriceps exercises in detail because these plus active movement of the toes can also be done by a patient with a fractured leg in a plaster of Paris to keep the muscles in trim. The quadriceps are the massive group of muscles in the front of the thigh which straighten the knee. After an injury to the knee they soon weaken and waste considerably. Building these muscles up again through exercises is essential for full recovery to occur. The easiest way to learn them is to go along to your physiotherapy department and ask them to show you how it is done. Most hospital departments are only too willing to teach you things if only you *ask*.

Method of teaching quadriceps exercises. Ask your patient to tighten up the muscles in the front of the thigh. If it is done correctly he should be able to feel the quadriceps contracting with his own hand. You can test the contraction by holding the patella. If the quadriceps are relaxed the patella can be 'wobbled' from side to side. If they are contracted it is rigid. Ask the patient to continue this tightening, pushing the knee downwards and at the same time dorsiflexing the foot. After a few moments he can relax and then do the exercise all over again, continuing for five to ten minutes several times a day. Once used to that he can try lifting the leg upwards as well (straight-leg raising). After a week of these exercises most patients will feel a noticeable improvement.

Crutches

Today the handing out of crutches requires a little more finesse than in the days of Long John Silver. Sound and sturdy crutches must be supplied with rubbers on the ends which have plenty of tread left. Both must match and be checked for loose fittings. If they are axillary crutches they should reach from about 8 cm (3 in) below the axilla to the floor approximately 24 cm (9 in) from the foot. If they are elbow crutches, the hand grips should be at a height such that the elbow is slightly bent.

A very important point about the use of the axillary crutches is that no weight at all is placed on the top pad. This pad is there only to be pressed into the side of the chest for stability. All the weight is taken by the hands on the grips.

Next, let the patient get used to the feel of the crutches and stand still balancing. Show the patient how to walk, standing close by all the time in case of falling. If he is partial weight-bearing make him take small steps keeping the crutches in line with the 'bad' leg. If non-weight-bearing, he should place both crutches just a little in front of the feet and swing through up to them. In the case of a long leg plaster he will have to hitch up the hip on the affected side so that the plaster will clear the floor. With below-knee supports the knee is just bent.

Warn the patient that at home there will be carpets and uneven surfaces which are a danger; it is best to ask a member of the family to stand by while he walks for the first day, just in case a fall occurs. I always ask the patient when he first has crutches not to try going up stairs with them at least for several days; it is just too dangerous! Edging up on the bottom, although undignified, is safe.

A final point concerns standing and sitting. Ask your patient to reverse until the chair can be felt against the legs, then transfer both crutches to one hand, hold onto the chair with the other and sit slowly.

MUSCULAR INJURIES

During sports and some other activities, muscle fibres can be torn and bleeding may occur either into the muscle itself or between muscles. When bleeding is inside the muscle, the blood remains localized as a haematoma, whereas when bleeding is between the muscles it can also track up and down the leg between the fascia. Treatment is first to exclude any bony injury, then to apply a firm support to the part and let the patient rest. When he is at home, advise elevation of the affected limb. If possible apply cold, maybe in the form of ice in a plastic bag, over the affected part for a while, as this helps to stop bleeding. It is wrong for the patient to attempt any exercises for about a week until the acute phase is over.

Muscle tendons also frequently tear. A common injury is to the achilles tendon which can be easily felt above the heel. Only a minor force is required to rupture it especially in the older patient. Classically, the patient is unable to stand on the toes.

9 Upper limb, spinal column and facial injuries

THE UPPER LIMB

When dealing with injuries of the upper limb there are a few general points of care which I would like to mention before dealing with the individual injuries. It is easy for the inexperienced to underestimate the amount of severe pain which these injuries can bring. The fingertips especially can be very sensitive, injuries to them sending huge labourers fainting to the floor. The lesson is, therefore, to have your patient lying down if he is in severe pain. Thus he will not faint and will be able to cope with what may be a long delay before final treatment.

All rings and bracelets must be removed from an arm or hand before the swelling becomes severe. Even the short time that a patient is in the x-ray department is enough to make a ring need to be cut off. If a ring is to be removed, try the simple methods first. Easiest of all is to smear soap all over the finger and under the ring. Stand in front of the patient and grasp the edge of the ring with the index and middle fingers of both your hands; you need short strong nails for this (Fig. 77). While you pull on the ring, massage the skin and push the bulge under the ring bit by bit with your thumbs. There are two other methods which you may be interested in, but I do not think that they are likely to succeed if the first method fails unless your fingernails have not been able to grip correctly. The first is to wrap stout twine round the finger from the tip up towards the ring. The end of the twine is then passed under the ring. You then unwind the twine while applying traction on it towards the finger tip. Alternatively, a piece of fine tape is soaped and passed under the ring, then both ends are circled round and round the finger while being pulled; this will occasionally do the trick. Most women feel that rings are something special and to some they are items of extreme sentimental value; their removal can occasionally be a tragedy. The final method, cutting, must therefore be only a last resort (Fig. 78).

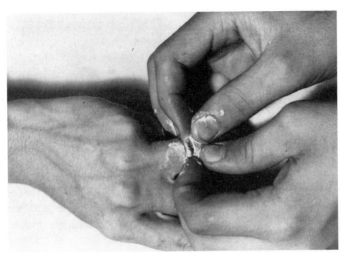

Fig. 77. *The easiest way to remove a tight ring is to pull on it with your fingernails while massaging the skin through it using the thumbs.*

With all injuries to the arm or shoulder, remember to check the circulation, movements and sensations to the limb when the patient first arrives. The patient must be undressed adequately before the doctor examines him, so that both sides of the body can be compared. The doctor must also be able to see not only, for example, the injured wrist, but also the elbow and shoulder on the same side. With a severe fracture it may take as many as three nurses to get the patient undressed without damaging the clothing or hurting the patient. Strangely enough, some footballers will go through considerable pain to keep the club football jersey in one piece and will stubbornly resist any attempt to cut it.

FRACTURES OF THE CLAVICLE

Clavicle fracture is at times seen accompanying fractures of the ribs in road traffic accident victims, but it is usually found in children and young adults following a fall on the shoulder or outstretched arm.

Although the clavicle is quite a small bone, the patient very frequently looks as 'white as a ghost' and feels faint. In most instances the diagnosis can be made as the patient walks in through the door clutching his arm in the characteristic way.

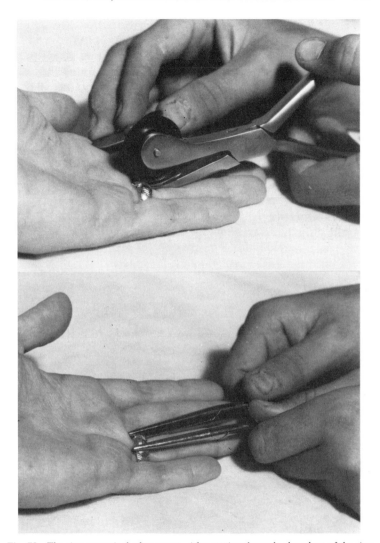

Fig. 78. *The ring cutter is the last resort. After cutting through, the edges of the ring must be separated with two heavy artery forceps. If the ring is heavy this may be the most difficult part.*

Sit your patient down until you have removed clothes to the waist. To remove a jersey, for instance, first bring it up to the armpits while someone holds onto the arm on the affected side. The good arm is then removed and the jersey gently brought over the head. Finally, it is brought down over the injured side and the arm held firmly by the elbow, while the jersey is pulled over the forearm and hand. Temporary support can then be given by the use of a triangular sling with a substantial pad around the neck. Final treatment will consist of either continuing the sling in comparatively trivial cases or using some form of bandage to keep the shoulders pulled backwards. One method shown in Fig. 79 is called the figure-of-eight bandage. The patient sits on a stool and the nurse stands behind. Ask the patient to put the hands on the hips and draw the shoulders back. Padding is applied over the shoulders and in the axillae. The bandages are then applied while the nurse, with the knee in the patient's back, keeps the shoulders drawn backwards. A sling is then sometimes applied. This manoeuvre, although correcting the deformity, can cause the patient severe pain and should be carried out gently. After application, check once again the circulation, movements and sensations to the arms.

Warn the patient of problems which may occur, such as 'digging in' at the axilla causing pins and needles in the fingers and show

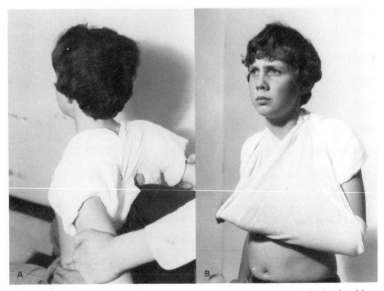

Fig. 79. A, *A figure-of-eight bandage or its equivalent is applied while the shoulders are drawn back;* **B**, *a sling then completes the treatment.*

how 'easing' the bandage with the fingers can help to stop this. Tightening the bandages daily may be required at first and your patient may find it advisable to wear loose baggy clothing over the top of the bandage and sling.

DISLOCATION OF THE SHOULDER

Again, another very common injury, dislocation of the shoulder is most often seen in young adult rugby or football players who are tackled and fall onto the shoulder, or in old ladies who stumble. The features are fairly straight forward in a normal-sized patient, but in the obese, diagnosis can occasionally cause problems. The points to note when diagnosing a dislocation (Fig. 80) are:

1. The shoulder is angulated instead of curved
2. The centre line of the humerus does not run through the joint
3. Sometimes the head of humerus can be felt anteriorly

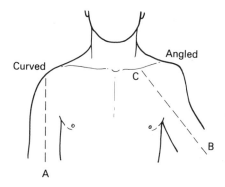

Fig. 80. *A dislocated left shoulder. Note that the shoulder is angulated; line B does not run through the joint whereas line A does; and the head of the humerus can sometimes be felt at point C.*

The patient will probably arrive clutching the arm as with a fractured clavicle. Sit or lie the patient down, depending on the severity of the pain. One of the positions in Fig. 81 will be most comfortable:

1. Lying on the back on a trolley, with the backrest slightly raised and the elbow supported on a pillow.

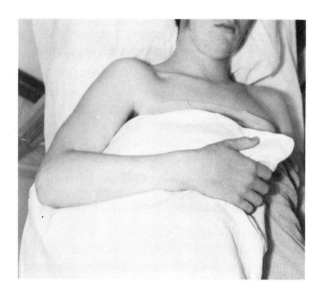

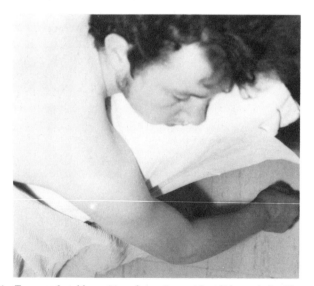

Fig. 81. *Two comfortable positions for patients with a dislocated shoulder or other arm injury.*

2. Sitting in a chair wearing a sling or holding the arm.
3. Lying face down on a trolley with a pillow under the chest, while the arm hangs straight down. Spontaneous reduction occasionally occurs in this position if the patient is relaxed.

Drugs such as pethidine have a tendency to make some patients feel as though they are 'floating in the air' and frequently others vomit. Therefore, if such drugs are given it is sensible to have the patient laying down. Before anything else is done, check the circulation, movements and sensations to the arm.

Reduction may be under a general anaesthetic, pethidine and diazepam or Entonox, or nothing may be given depending on the patient and the skill of the operator. There are two main methods. Firstly, the 'Hippocratic', where the operator takes off a shoe and places the foot in the patient's armpit. While doing this the doctor then applies traction to the arm. Another method more commonly employed is Kocher's. With this, the doctor will apply traction to the arm with the elbow at right angles. The arm is rotated externally and abducted and then, while still externally rotated, adducted across the chest. Finally, if the arm is internally rotated, the joint usually slips easily back into position. During both of these manoeuvres the nurse may be asked to press over the head of the humerus or apply counter-traction round the armpit.

Nothing is more infuriating than to get the shoulder reduced and then have it slip out again when the patient is awakening from the anaesthetic. Abduction is the movement which is most likely to cause this, so after reduction stay by the side of your patient and keep the arm against his side. An arm sling is applied, with a small piece of gamgee in the armpit to prevent intertrigo. The whole is then bound to the chest wall with crêpe or Netalast to prevent abduction (Fig. 82).

DISLOCATED ACROMIOCLAVICULAR JOINT

The acromioclavicular joint may be either subluxated or completely dislocated, giving the shoulder a characteristic and unusual look (Fig. 83). Pain is sometimes severe at first, but should not require strong analgesics. Treatment varies; for example, the arm on the affected side may just be supported in an arm sling or a more

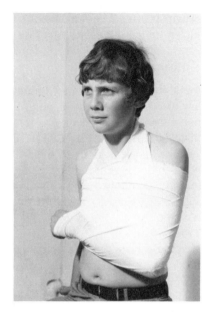

Fig. 82. *After the dislocated shoulder has been reduced, the arm is held to the side with a sling and then bound well to the chest.*

complex form of bandaging, where adhesive strapping encircles the shoulder and elbow, may be used. This presses down on felt pads over the outer end of the clavicle and under the elbow (Fig. 84).

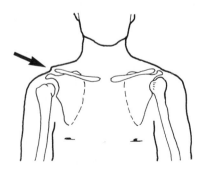

Fig. 83. *The characteristic 'step' on the shoulder seen in patients with a dislocated acromioclavicular joint.*

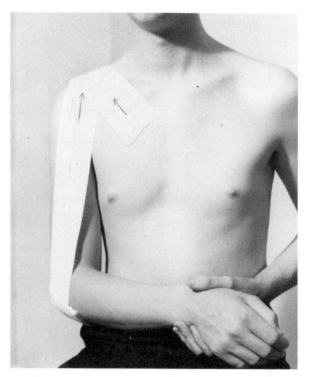

Fig. 84. *One of many treatments for a dislocated acromioclavicular joint.*

FRACTURES OF THE UPPER END OF THE HUMERUS

Fractures of the humerus (Fig. 85) are most common in the elderly and young children. An old lady trips or blacks out, falling onto her outstretched hand or onto her shoulder. Even though on the radiograph the fracture may look very bad, conservative treatment is normally all that is required; few patients will require a formal reduction under general anaesthesia. When the patient arrives, undress her carefully to see if she has injured any other part of the body during the fall. Test the circulation, movements and sensations to the limb. Ask her carefully *why* she fell and bear in mind such conditions as a minor cerebrovascular accident, epilepsy, Stokes-Adams attacks and failing eyesight.

Treatment will obviously vary with the specific fracture, but a fairly common approach is to apply a pad to the axilla, put the arm

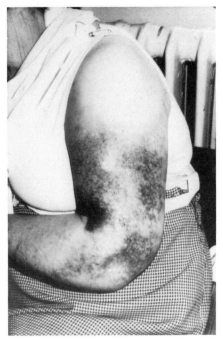

Fig. 85. *The characteristic bruising which accompanies a fracture of the upper end of the humerus. Blood tracks down beneath the deltoid muscle and shows as bruising round the elbow.*

in a sling and bind it to the chest wall as with a dislocation; occasionally a large roll is required (Fig. 86) to aid reduction. The shoulder joint, especially in the elderly, is very prone to become stiff if immobilized for any length of time. Because of this the

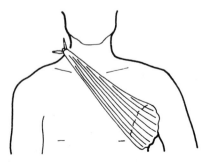

Fig. 86. *Sometimes a large pad is needed to keep the fracture reduced. This can be placed in tube-gauze and tied round the neck to keep it in position.*

binding to the chest wall will be short-lived; later, gentle swinging exercises can be started. By three weeks, immobilization should have been discontinued and the patient should be actively moving the arm to get shoulder movements back. Your patient must never be allowed home until you are sure that she will be able to cope with the injury. Ask if she has someone at home to look after her; if not, inquire into the social background. Is she stable on her feet and capable of getting in and out of bed and to the toilet?

FRACTURES OF THE SHAFT OF THE HUMERUS

Shaft fractures occur most commonly in the 20–40-year-old age group and are not as common as those in the last section. The bones tend to be 'wobbly' and displacement severe. Although checking the circulation, movements and sensations is essential, the most common positive finding is damage to the radial nerve where it winds round the shaft of the humerus (Fig. 87). Initially,

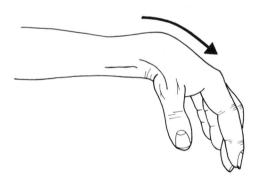

Fig. 87. *Drop wrist is commonly produced by damage to the radial nerve when it winds round the shaft of the humerus.*

the patient will be more comfortable sitting up on a trolley with a collar and cuff sling applied. This allows the arm to hang, thus applying traction to the distal fragment and easing the pain a little.

A huge problem arises if the patient is a struggling unconscious head injury. One frequently sees the fractured arm waved about bending in all directions. If this happens, ask one nurse to hold on to the arm and do nothing else. Ensure that the circulation is still intact, then quickly apply temporary splints to the arm, based on the method described in the next paragraph.

The three-splint method

With a cooperative and sedated patient, a general anaesthetic may be unnecessary for splinting. The patient should sit on the side of the trolley with legs dangling over the side; never use a chair because the patient may faint with the discomfort and you will then have a considerable problem. Thinking ahead about what might happen is one of the cornerstones of good accident and emergency technique. A collar-and-cuff sling is applied with the elbow at a right angle and orthopaedic wool is wrapped round the upper arm and elbow (Fig. 88). Three splints are then measured and padded. The first goes from just below the fold of the skin in the axilla down to just above the bend in the elbow. It is essential that this one in particular is not too long, otherwise it can dig in causing pressure sores or affect the blood supply to the limb. The second splint is placed more posteriorly, while the third and largest is on the outside extending from the elbow up to the shoulder. During the application of the splints, gentle downwards traction is

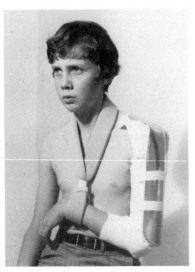

Fig. 88. *The three-splint method of treating a fracture of the shaft of the humerus.*

applied on the arm while an assistant straps them together. The whole is then bandaged in position and the circulation, movements and sensations once again tested.

The Bohler U plaster slab method

The preparation of the patient is the same as for the three-splint method. A 15 cm slab of plaster is then measured to extend from the top of the shoulder, round the elbow to a point on the lower arm below the armpit (Fig. 89). This is held in place by an encircling moistened cotton bandage. There are other minor variations of this plaster.

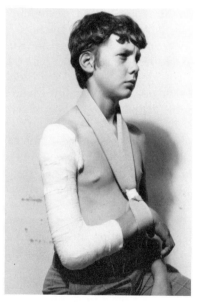

Fig. 89. *The Bohler U plaster slab method of treating a fracture of the neck of the humerus. As with the splint method, gentle traction is applied to the bent arm while the plaster is being applied so that the bones are brought into alignment.*

With both methods, remember that the arm will not stay as you see it; bleeding from fractures is progressive, increasing the swelling. With the splintage making an unyielding cylinder, this will further increase the swelling and cause oedema around the elbow. Bearing this in mind, your patient should always return the next day to assess the progress. If patients are simply sent home with a fracture clinic appointment, some will suffer immense pain and discomfort until the date of the next appointment, rather than worry the hospital staff with an intermediate visit.

SUPRACONDYLAR FRACTURES OF THE HUMERUS

A supracondylar fracture of the humerus is commonly seen in children. If it is displaced and requires reduction the patient must always be kept in hospital to ensure that the circulation is satisfactory. On arrival the child must be laid on a trolley and will probably be most comfortable with a pad under the elbow and the forearm resting on the abdomen. Cut off clothing unless you think that it is merely an undisplaced crack fracture. The child will be crying or very upset, and pale with the pain. Keep the parent by the child's side so that he or she can be seen at all times; in most cases this, plus a confident, reassuring and friendly attitude, will help to settle the child down considerably. Make it the task of one nurse to feel for the radial pulse on the affected side every 15 minutes.

With these fractures a very serious condition called Volkmann's ischaemic contracture can occur. If the ends of the fractured bone have damaged the brachial artery or made it go into spasm (Fig. 90) there will obviously be signs which you should notice, that is, skin changes and a diminished or absent pulse. This was mentioned in some detail in Chapter 8. There may, however, be enough of a collateral circulation for the hand to stay alive, but there will not be enough blood to supply the muscles of the forearm. When this occurs the muscles will 'shrivel' up and be replaced gradually by fibrous tissue, making the fingers and hand grotesquely contracted. By the time this has occurred, it is too late to save the muscles. However, early warning signs do occur and the nurse must be on the alert for them. These are firstly all the signs and symptoms of an impaired circulation as previously mentioned *plus* an inability to extend the fingers; this is accompanied by severe pain in the forearm if you try to extend the fingers passively.

You should summon senior orthopaedic help immediately. The doctor will first want any cast or splint which is applied to be either

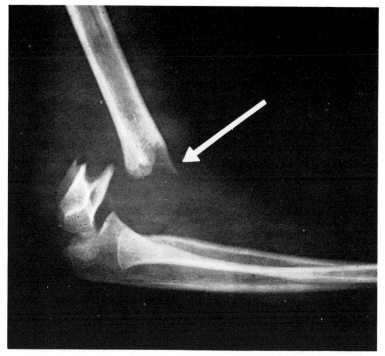

Fig. 90. *A radiograph showing a supracondylar fracture of the humerus. The arrow points to a sharp edge of fractured bone which could damage a blood vessel.*

removed completely or cut through right down to the skin. If you are asked to split a cast because the limb has a poor circulation, it is vital that the underlying padding and stockinette is divided; merely cutting the plaster is of no use at all. If this does not help, urgent operation will be required.

Treatment

If the fracture is undisplaced all that is required is a collar-and-cuff sling, with the elbow higher up than the usual right angle. If displaced, a general anaesthetic will be necessary. The doctor will manipulate the arm carefully, feeling the radial pulse frequently to ensure that the circulation is unimpaired. The arm will be held in a collar-and-cuff sling once again and should be stable. Some

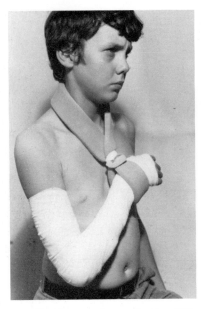

Fig. 91. *Some supracondylar fractures also require the addition of plaster of Paris slab.*

doctors, however, prefer in addition a posterior plaster slab running from the wrist to the shoulder (Fig. 91).

It will be noticed that there is often a great deal of swelling following this fracture, or indeed any serious injury round the elbow. This is because the tissues round the elbow are very elastic, allowing fluid freedom to move. Because of this, never have any non-yielding material completely encircling an injured elbow; it is asking for trouble.

DISLOCATION OF THE ELBOW

From a purely nursing point of view the care of a supracondylar fracture and that of a dislocated elbow (Fig. 92) are very similar indeed. The same dangers with the circulation are evident, but to a lesser degree. Observations, however, must be just as relentless. Reduction is once again under a general anaesthetic and afterwards the elbow will simply be kept in a collar-and-cuff sling. As long as the circulation is satisfactory the patient will probably be

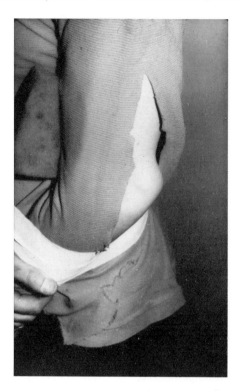

Fig. 92. *The typical presentation of a dislocated elbow.*

allowed home afterwards. As a final point, there is a simple way of differentiating the supracondylar fracture from the dislocated elbow. An imaginary triangle is drawn between the two epicondyles of the humerus and the olecranon. With a fracture all three points are in the same vertical plane whereas with a dislocation the triangle is at an angle.

PULLED ELBOW

The classical picture here is of a toddler being either swung by the parents or lifted, so that traction occurs to the extended arm (Fig. 93). The action presumably pulls the head of the radius momentarily away from the ligament which holds it to the side of the ulna. You are presented with a child who will not use the affected arm; it

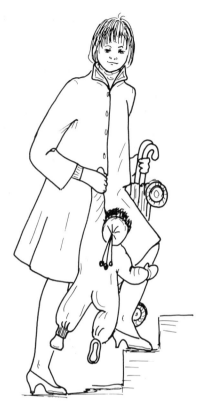

Fig. 93. *The classic way for a small child to get a 'pulled elbow'.*

just hangs still at the side. Twisting the forearm or touching the site of the injury will produce crying. Be sure to have the whole of the arm exposed so that the doctor can examine it all and compare it with the good side. He will have to feel and move all the joints watching the child's reaction to locate the tender area.

Treatment

Treatment is sometimes hardly necessary; often the movements involved in having a radiograph are sufficient to relocate the radius. If not, the doctor will supinate the forearm while flexing the elbow. Afterwards, the arm is kept in a sling for a day or so (if the child allows it). Pain may disappear immediately or settle gradually over the next few days.

FRACTURES OF THE HEAD OF THE RADIUS

Apart from tenderness over the site, the main feature of fracture of the radial head is pain on pronating and supinating the forearm. From the point of view of the nurse there is little that is specific to say about it. Sometimes the fracture is so difficult to see on the radiograph that it can be missed if the doctor is not meticulous. A reasonable amount of swelling usually occurs during the first 24 hours, but this seldom causes any problems. A collar-and-cuff sling is all that is required in the majority of cases (Fig. 94).

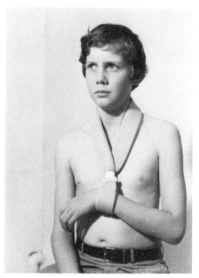

Fig. 94. *The standard collar-and-cuff sling.*

FRACTURES OF THE FOREARM

Forearm fracture is quite a common injury, especially in children where the greenstick variety is frequently seen. Displacement of the bones can either be non-existent in the case of minor cracks or range right up the scale to the 'swan-neck' deformity shown in Fig.

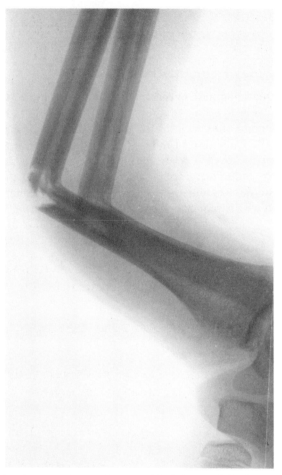

Fig. 95. *A radiograph showing fracture of both bones of the forearm; they are angled at 90°, making a 'swan-neck' deformity.*

95. Even in the worst cases the patient usually walks into the department. He must be cared for at once, laid on a trolley with the backrest raised a little, and the arm well supported with pillows, sandbags or foam blocks. It is rare for a sling to be comfortable when the patient is lying down. Minor cases can be assessed quickly, have a sling applied and then be asked to wait.

Warn all patients who may have a fracture not to let anything pass their lips. Even in these enlightened days there are many people who do not understand this rule. To some people it is kindness to offer the sick a drink. Also do not fall into the trap of saying 'don't have anything to eat before your anaesthetic'. I will never forget the old lady in the waiting room, who, after a four-hour wait for a general anaesthetic, said 'Will I have time for a second cup?' while holding onto her little flask!

As with all fractures check the circulation, movements and sensations to the limb at intervals. Pins and needles are common, as is slight circulatory impairment. However, even with severe deformities, serious problems are rare. If a limb has to be moved at all, for instance in x-ray, support it securely above and below the fracture site with your hands. If this is done with care and the patient has confidence in you, it will be almost painless. Surprisingly, it is fairly easy to get the clothing off in the majority of instances. Cutting is sometimes required, but with two people helping you most problems can be overcome.

Treatment

If undisplaced, the fracture will simply be immobilized in a long arm plaster and a sling applied to take the weight. If displaced, reduction under general anaesthetic will be required in almost every instance.

After manipulation. The patient must be in a good position if the plaster is to be applied easily, lying near the edge of the trolley, with the arm abducted; the elbow must be at right angles and the whole arm supported in the air by the fingers. It also helps to avoid too tight a plaster if the little finger is left free and the arm supported by the others (Fig. 96). The degree of rotation of the forearm will vary with the level of the fracture and the surgeon will probably want to mould the plaster to an oval shape to prevent movement of the bones. An x-ray image intensifier (Fig. 97) is invaluable in this sort of work, displaced fractures of both the radius and ulna being notoriously difficult to reduce. Even with this aid, problems still occur and plating of the radius is fairly often required.

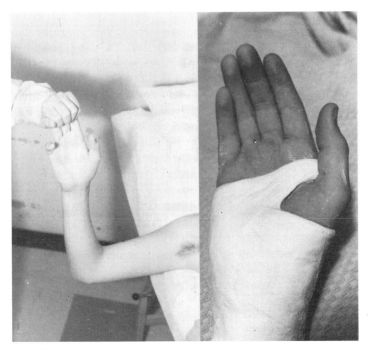

Fig. 96. *Before a long arm plaster is applied the patient is best positioned near the edge of the table.* **A**, *Hold the arm by the fingers and thumb, leaving the little finger free so that the plaster will not be too tight.* **B**, *The final level of the plaster over the palm of the hand.*

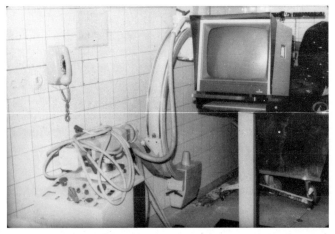

Fig. 97. *An x-ray image intensifier.*

COLLES' FRACTURE

Colles' fracture is one of the best known and most common fractures. Looking at one from the front, the hand is displaced towards the 'thumb' side (see Fig. 100); looking at it from the side (lateral view), the hand is pushed upwards making the arm look like a dinner fork (Fig. 98). The fracture commonly occurs in elderly ladies who have a simple fall and put their hands out to save themselves. Most of the patients are still able to move their arm about quite easily because the bone ends are 'rammed' together (impacted). The majority of cases are not associated with any other injury, except perhaps bruising of the elbow which shows up days later and can worry the patient.

X-ray changes

I would like to describe the changes shown on the radiograph in a little detail, because they serve as a very useful starter to you in your study of x-ray films. Fig. 99(a) shows the normal lateral view of the wrist. If you draw a straight line through points A and B of

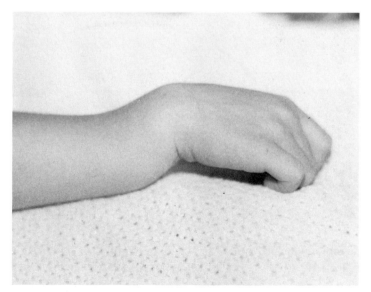

Fig. 98. *A fracture of the lower end of the radius with the typical 'dinner fork' deformity.*

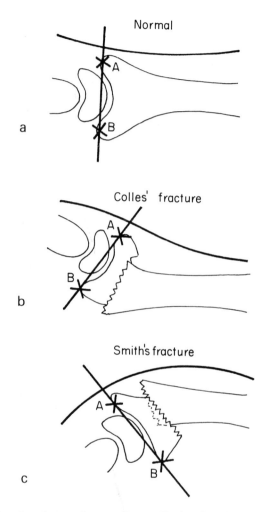

Fig. 99. (**a**) *A lateral view of a normal wrist. The line through points A and B is upright or tilts only a few degrees anteriorly. If the same line is drawn through a Colles' (**b**) or Smith's (**c**) fracture, it will be tilted posteriorly or anteriorly respectively, as shown.*

the radius you will notice that it is upright. A Colles' fracture occurs in the lower 2–3 cm of the radius, tilting this line backwards (Fig. 99b). As well as tilting, there is an upwards (posterior) displacement of the distal fragment along with a degree of

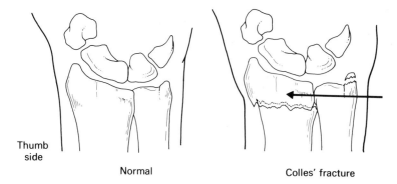

Thumb
side

Normal   Colles' fracture

Fig. 100. *A drawing taken from a radiograph of the wrist, showing how the whole hand is displaced towards the thumb in cases of Colles' fracture.*

impaction. Looking at the front view of the wrist (Fig. 100) the radius is seen to be displaced towards the thumb, carrying the hand with it. Sometimes a little peg of bone is also pulled off the ulna (ulna styloid).

Treatment

Any rings are removed from the fingers before swelling makes them too tight. You must find out why the patient fell, to ensure that he does not have a medical condition. If a general anaesthetic is to be given ask if he has any tablets from the doctor and also enquire into any past illnesses. This is all essential information for the anaesthetist. Although reduction under general anaesthesia is the most common course, this is not the only method which can be employed, others are:

1. Local injection of 1% lignocaine into the fracture haematoma from the dorsum of the wrist.
2. Diazepam and pethidine given following one another intravenously are quite effective in many instances.
3. Regional nerve block. Lignocaine is injected into the sheath of the brachial plexus either in the neck or, more commonly, in the upper medial part of the upper arm. A wait of about 20 minutes is then required until anaesthesia is complete.
4. Regional anaesthesia. The arm is elevated for a few minutes and then a sphygmomanometer cuff is applied to the upper

arm and inflated to prevent arterial flow. Bupivacaine 0.5% is then injected intravenously (about 20 ml) causing a mottling of the skin of the affected arm. After about 20 minutes, as the arm becomes anaesthetized, another cuff similarly inflated is placed just below the first. When this is done the first is then removed. The second cuff therefore lies against an anaesthetized part of the arm and is more comfortable for the patient.

After the reduction the cuff is slowly released. Two doctors are required, one will be an anaesthetist, who will have the sole responsibility for looking after the block and the other will care for the fracture. Fatalities have occurred! Full resuscitation equipment must be available during this procedure in case uncontrollable fits occur. It is the nurse's responsibility, in addition to helping both doctors, to keep an eye on the cuff pressure to ensure that it does not fall.

At the time of writing, this method of anaesthesia is under government review and could well be banned in the future.

The reduction itself usually entails initial traction on the arm to disimpact the bone ends, which must be done with the elbow at right angles so that there is no traction on the nerves. This is followed by the doctor pushing directly down over the distal fragment with the heel of the hand and simultaneously pressing the hand over to the ulna side of the arm. While the doctor holds the arm in this position, the nurse applies the plaster slab, or splints, and bandages it into position. If splints are being applied they are measured as shown in Fig. 101, the upper one from the knuckles to

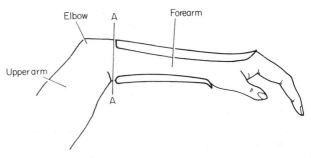

Fig. 101. *The measurement of splints for a case of Colles' fracture. Stop at point A so that the elbow can still bend.*

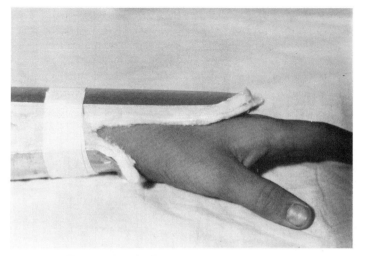

Fig. 102. *Details of the lower end of Colles' splints.*

point A and the lower one from the bend in the wrist to point A. The end of the lower splint at the wrist is curved under and its edge near the thumb eased over so that movements of a swollen thumb will not cause a sore (Fig. 102). Some like the splint to be left straight and others prefer the top one to be bent and twisted into the same position as the plaster slab. Initially, the patient is allowed to wear a sling, but the next day when the patient returns for a splint or plaster check this should be removed and more movements encouraged. If a plaster slab was applied in the first instance it will require converting into a short arm plaster, unless swelling is troublesome, in which case the patient will have to return daily until it can be safely completed (Fig. 103).

Give your patient advice to prevent or remove swelling after reduction of the fracture. Cutting or loosening the plaster should be a rarity if these rules are followed:

1. Never have the arm hanging down
2. If walking around, either keep the arm in the sling (in the first 24 hours) or walk with it by your chest
3. When sitting down at home have it resting high up on the arm of a chair on cushions (Fig. 104)
4. Work hard at active movements of the fingers at every available opportunity

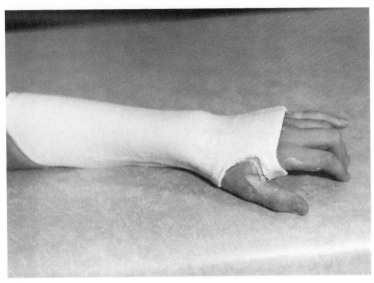

Fig. 103. *A plaster back slab for Colles' fracture.*

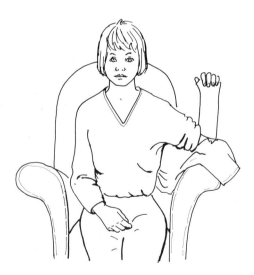

Fig. 104. *When the patient is sitting at home the injured arm should rest high up on cushions on the arm of a chair. This will aid venous return far more than if the arm is kept in a sling.*

Items 3 and 4, done for two hours, will bring considerable relief even to cases with severe swelling.

A Colles' fracture is rather prone to slipping out of position again. To check on this possibility the doctor will probably want your patient to be reviewed within about a week of the reduction. The splint or plaster will be worn for approximately six weeks.

SMITH'S FRACTURE

Smith's fracture is similar to Colles' fracture except for the following points. It is caused by a fall on the back of the wrist pushing the bone ends downwards (anteriorly). This is shown in Fig. 99(c). Notice that the line AB is now in the opposite position to that shown for a Colles' fracture. The importance of the fracture is in its similarity to Colles' fracture. If the doctor does not notice the difference and tries to reduce it in the same way as a Colles' fracture, disaster will result. Be on the alert, mistakes do happen!

Immobilization is by a full arm plaster with the wrist supinated. There are no specific extra nursing points.

FRACTURE OF THE SCAPHOID

The scaphoid is a tiny bone in the wrist, in what is called the 'anatomical snuff-box' (Fig. 105). It is quite frequently fractured, giving pain and tenderness in this snuff-box. The fracture, however, has a very unusual habit of not showing up on radiographs taken just after the injury. If, because of this, the fracture is missed, the bone may give trouble in later life, leaving the patient with a permanently painful and weak wrist. So you see, despite its small size, this bone can cause severe problems. Can you think of an occupation where having a weak wrist does not matter?

To get over this problem, if anyone is tender in this snuff-box, even if the radiograph shows nothing, that patient is treated as though there is a fracture. This will mean the application of a plaster. Then after 10 days it is radiographed again without plaster; after this time the fracture line will show up more clearly. As with a Colles' fracture, the plaster will be worn for about six weeks. If union is not complete, however, it may have to be re-applied.

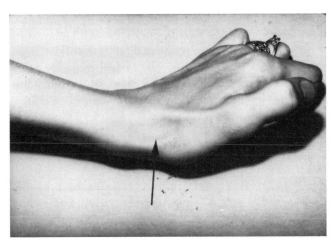

Fig. 105. *The anatomical snuff-box.*

TENOSYNOVITIS

This condition, which is most commonly seen in the back of the wrist but also commonly occurs in the foot, is an inflammation of the sheath in which a tendon runs. Its main cause is a period of excessive use of the part involved. One of the fascinating features of it is the 'crackling' which can be felt under the skin when the affected tendons are used. Treatment is by immobilization of the surrounding joints until the condition settles.

BENNETT FRACTURE

Bennett fracture is an oblique fracture through the base of the thumb metacarpal and involving the joint surface. As with a scaphoid fracture, it usually occurs in fairly young adults.

Reduction is usually required and sometimes needs general anaesthesia, although with minimal displacement Entonox is effective. The base of the thumb requires extra protection with felt to prevent sores occurring after reduction and plastering. If reduction is not successful, an operation will be required.

FRACTURES OF THE METACARPALS

The skin on the back of the hand is very loose and therefore swelling occurs readily after injury, in direct contrast to the palm which has a tough unyielding sheet of fascia discouraging swelling. With fractures of the metacarpals, therefore, most of the swelling will be on the back of the hand. The most common injury is a fracture of the neck of the little finger. This is invariably caused by the patient punching someone or something or, very rarely, by falling onto the knuckle. Schoolboys and young men make up 99 per cent of the patients.

Treatment varies with individual doctors. Even if nothing is done to reduce the displaced fracture quite a reasonable functional result is obtained. If displacement is only slight, the finger can be supported on a splint. If it is markedly displaced, most would attempt reduction under either general or local anaesthesia. The method is shown in Fig. 106. After reduction the finger is splinted as mentioned above or held in the flexed position over a bandage (Fig. 107).

Other fractures of the metacarpals are, in the main, of the shafts of the bones. Few require reduction. Immobilization varies from a simple crêpe bandage type of support, to the finger splint mentioned earlier or a full hand splint. All these methods also have their plaster equivalents.

As a rule most people with hand injuries will walk with the hand at the side, unless pain is severe when he will walk with it across the chest. Try to encourage the patient to keep it high; this will ease swelling and take away most of the throbbing pain that is

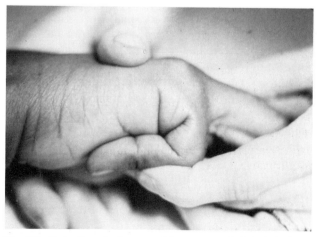

Fig. 106. *Reduction of a fracture of the metacarpal of the little finger.*

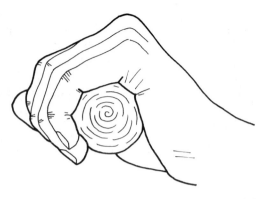

Fig. 107. *Fingers over a bandage, a method sometimes used to immobilize fractures.*

frequently found. If the injury is severe a triangular sling will be necessary, but, as mentioned with a Colles' fracture, getting the arm out of the sling and elevated on pillows is far better.

FRACTURES OF THE PHALANGES

Fractures of the phalanges are perhaps the most important fractures in this chapter. To understand why, get an elastic band and fix your thumb to the palm of the hand so that it cannot move. Try to write, eat, dress yourself or hold a bandage. Now do you understand what I mean? So very small, yet so important.

The majority of phalangeal fractures involve the bones of the tips of the fingers (terminal phalanges). These injuries occur when the fingers are trapped, for instance, in a door or machinery (Fig. 108). Pain is severe because there is little space for bleeding to spread so the finger throbs a lot. Sometimes the pulp space of the finger is so tense with haematoma under pressure that the tip looks ischaemic. Another presentation of the blood is posteriorly under the nail (subungual haematoma) (Fig. 109). This should be released as shown in Fig. 110 by making a hole in the nail with a red-hot paper clip or with a fine drill (e.g. a Pendril); immediate relief of pain occurs and your patient will be very thankful. Alternatively a blade may be slid under the nail to release the blood (Fig. 111).

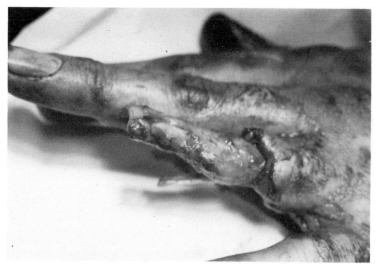

Fig. 108. *Severe 'degloving' injury caused by machinery.*

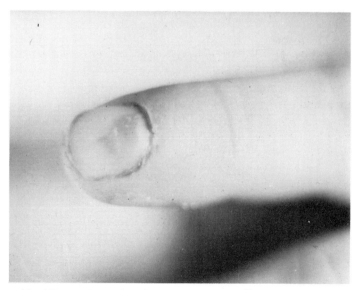

Fig. 109. *A subungual haematoma (a collection of blood under the nail).*

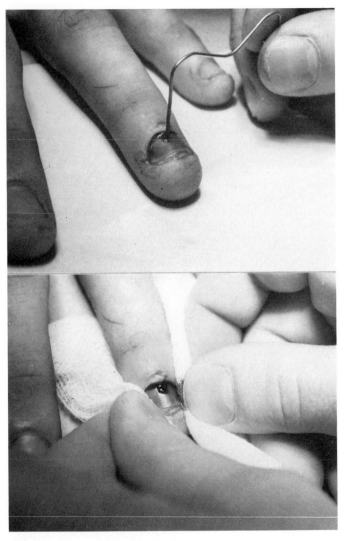

Fig. 110. *To release the blood a heated paperclip is pressed into the nail until it is felt to 'give'. The blood will then pour out naturally or can be helped by little gentle squeezing.*

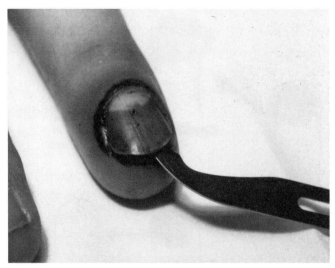

Fig. 111. *If the haematoma extends to the tip of the nail, a blade can simply be pushed up to release the blood. A local anaesthetic is not necessary and this procedure is far less frightening for the patient.*

Treatment

Most fractures require only cushioning with tube gauze against knocks. It is essential that this in no way constricts the finger since pain and bleeding will be increased. Advise your patient to keep the finger raised to ease any throbbing. The fractures are frequently compound, the wounds mainly occurring on the posterior of the finger round the nail. If the proximal part of the nail is flipped out on top of the skin, this part is best cut off with scissors so that exudate can drain freely (Fig. 112). A firmly attached nail is best left in place giving support and protection to the fracture. If, however, it is completely lifted off its bed or hanging on by a shred, remove it, otherwise the tissue underneath will soon be infected. When a nail is removed, ensure that all bleeding has been stopped before a dressing is applied. If this is not done it will bleed considerably into the dressing and then dry by the next day, making a rigid unyielding, smelling mass (Fig. 113). Dressing must be non-stick, either Melolin or a few layers of *tulle* or a combination of both. All of the above applies equally well to fingertip injuries where no fracture is found.

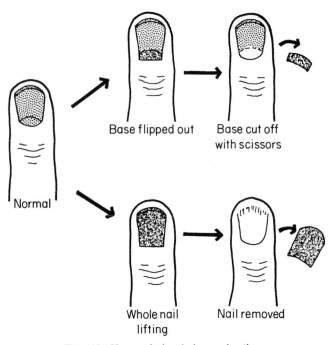

Fig. 112. *How to deal with damaged nails.*

Normal

Base flipped out

Base cut off with scissors

Whole nail lifting

Nail removed

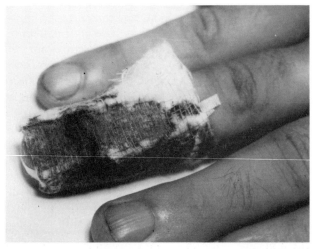

Fig. 113. *If bleeding has not stopped before the dressing is applied, this is the result the next day: a dressing which is as hard as rock because the blood has dried and which is painful to remove even after soaking.*

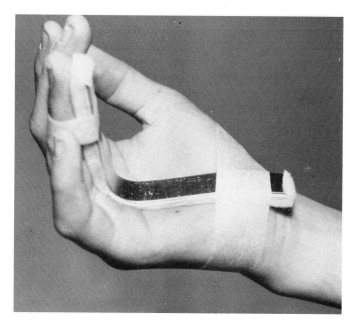

Fig. 114. *A standard type of finger splint. The metacarpal joint is flexed and interphalangeal joints extended.*

With fractures of the other phalanges (proximal and middle) treatment is by splintage of the individual finger (Fig. 114) usually on its own but sometimes with its partner. If the injury is fairly minor, the finger may simply be strapped to its partner for support; this will still allow gentle flexing exercises (Fig. 115).

MALLET FINGER

If the end of the finger is forcibly flexed, the tendon which extends the finger can sometimes be torn through or a flake of bone pulled off the terminal phalanx (Fig. 116). The end of the finger can then only be actively flexed. When it hangs down like this it looks a little like a mallet, hence the term 'mallet finger· Treatment is to hold the finger in the hyperextended position with one of several types of splint or plaster.

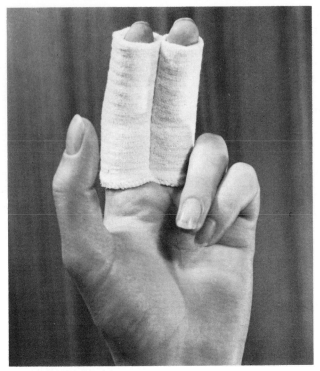

Fig. 115. *Bedford double finger stalls give support but allow movement.* (**With kind permission of Seton Products Ltd**)

THE SPINAL COLUMN

As with many topics in accident and emergency work, an in-depth study of spinal injuries would fill a book. Once again I am mentioning only the basics of the injuries themselves but balancing that with as much detail as I can on the initial nursing and treatment.

SIMPLE TORTICOLLIS

Torticollis is a very common condition, most of the patients being children. They wake up one morning to find the neck stiff, painful and twisted over to one side. A history of a previous injury is sometimes present. After x-ray, treatment is usually to support the neck in some form of collar (Fig. 117) until the condition subsides of its own accord. Analgesics in some form will be desirable. The care of the patient must not stop there, however; explanation must be given about the expected outcome and that it may take quite a while before the pain goes completely. Cold sprays to the affected muscles have their advocates, but I have yet to see any lasting effect.

CERVICAL DISC LESIONS

A condition which presents in a similar way, but in a far older age group, is prolapse of a cervical intervertebral disc. Pain is severe and travels down the arm to the fingers. Pins and needles and numbness can also occur. Initial treatment is similar, but ortho-

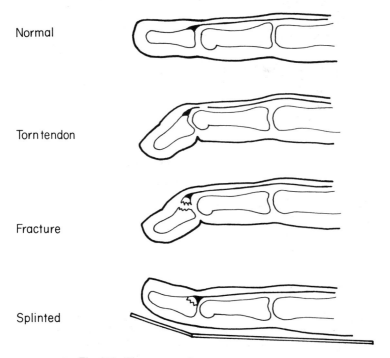

Normal

Torn tendon

Fracture

Splinted

Fig. 116. *The causes and treatment of mallet finger.*

paedic advice will then need to be sought. When sitting or lying, the patient will have to keep the head well supported to get relief.

WEDGE COMPRESSION FRACTURE

Looking from the side (lateral view), the bodies of the vertebrae are rectangular in shape. A very common fracture occurs round the middle of the back at T12–L1 level where the body of a vertebra is compressed, making it wedge-shaped (Fig. 118). With this fracture there is seldom any neurological involvement. However, a routine is essential if mistakes are to be prevented. Before you even start to move or undress the patient, ensure that he can feel and move the legs if the pain is central over the vertebrae. Even if all seems to be satisfactory, assume that the patient has a fracture until a radiograph proves otherwise. Handle

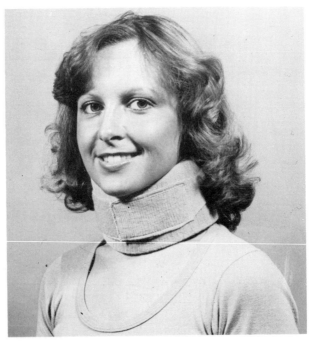

Fig. 117. *A simple and effective cervical collar.* (**With kind permission of Seton Products Ltd**)

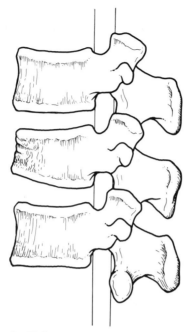

Fig. 118. *Wedge compression of a lumbar vertebra.*

the patient with utmost care, avoiding all spinal movements. Plenty of helpers may be required.

MAJOR SPINAL INJURIES

Suspicion that the patient may have a major spinal injury is of prime importance. Any patient who has had an injury to the head which is serious enough to cause unconsciousness has also had an injury which is serious enough to cause a fracture of the spinal column. Never forget the routine of asking the patient what happened or, if the patient is unconscious, of asking the ambulance men, *before the patient is moved or undressed.* A good history of the accident is often the only hint you may have of there being a spinal injury. Place the patient on an accident trolley so that x-rays can be taken without moving him, also ensure that there is a mattress of substantial thickness so that the patient does not get pressure sores.

Warn the patient to lie still and take care not to jar the trolley. Ensure that any nurse dealing with the patient knows exactly what is suspected and try to get only the most senior nurses to help you. Do any lifting of limbs very slowly and carefully. Remove clothes with utmost gentleness, cutting them if necessary to avoid excessive movement. A major nursing blunder would be to remove clothing over the head (Fig. 119) thereby flexing the neck. This is the most dangerous movement in a cervical spine injury. Plan all the tasks beforehand with the nurses concerned so that all fully understand exactly what movements you are trying to make. Always have in the front of your mind a mental picture of the tiny, delicate spinal cord and how easily it could be injured by its surrounding robust bony canal.

If the fracture or dislocation is in the cervical spine, prevent the head from moving by placing sandbags on either side or with a temporary collar or a Vac-Pac splint (Fig. 120). As a final precaution, a senior experienced nurse should stay with the patient at all times and:

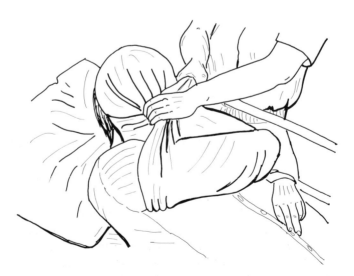

Fig. 119. *Removing clothes over the patient's head is dangerous with a cervical spine injury.*

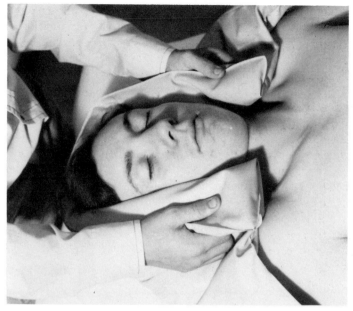

Fig. 120. *A Vac-Pac splint can be used for a spinal injury. It does, however, require very careful positioning.*

1. Ensure that no one nearby moves the patient
2. Ensure that the trolley is not knocked
3. Give the patient confidence that experienced help is always at hand
4. Watch constantly for deterioration, especially in cases of high cervical lesions where respirations may be seriously embarrassed as oedema of the cord and surrounding tissues progresses.

Radiographs should be taken on the accident trolley, preferably in the accident and emergency unit or in a nearby x-ray department so that no unnecessary movements occur. If the patient is moved, even the porters must be told what is wrong so that the patient has a smooth ride. Lateral views of the cervical spine should be the first to be taken; this will give the surgeon a fair idea of how much more movement to allow for other views. Patients with quadriplegia or paraplegia will then be transferred as soon as possible to a regional spinal injuries centre. Depending on the locality, transfer will be by very slow ambulance or even helicopter if this is available in the area.

It is pointless for the nurses in the spinal injury unit to turn the patient with care at regular intervals if, during a stay in the accident and emergency department, he has been motionless for hours on end. The damage will already have been done and pressure sores will show in a few days. Ensure from the outset that the patient is not lying in one position for more than two hours. Heels can be eased by placing a pillow under the calves (Fig. 121). Sacral pressure can be eased by wedges of foam under the patient

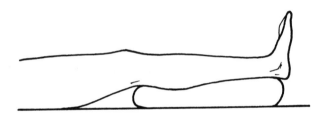

Fig. 121. *Very serious damage can be done to the pressure areas of a paraplegic patient while he waits in the accident and emergency department. Put a pillow under the calves.*

to move the weight around a little or by moving the skin around with the fingers, depending on the state of the fracture. If the patient's stay in the department is prolonged it may become necessary to intermittently catheterize the bladder to prevent bladder distention.

If the patient is not too badly injured elsewhere he will in all probability be immensely worried about his inability to feel or to move. No strict method of talking can be mentioned because the approach varies with every individual and the circumstances, but generally:

1. Do not lie, but perhaps hide the complete truth a little.
2. Remain encouraging, confident and reassuring. Leave the final news until the patient has been fully assessed at the spinal unit by experts in the field.

A final word of warning. Do not think of the spinal injury in isolation. Abdominal and chest trauma may be less obvious but may still be present.

ACUTE BACK STRAIN AND LUMBAR DISC LESIONS

Few patients with acute back strain and lumbar disc lesions attend the accident and emergency department.

The history is often of stooping, bending over or maybe lifting awkwardly. The back 'goes', becomes rigid and gives the patient very severe pain. Sometimes the patient is 'fixed' in one position and can only move with great difficulty. Never force your patient to lie down or sit, if it causes too much pain. You will often find that he will be happier leaning up against the trolley.

No 'cure' can be offered for these unfortunate patients in the short term. Treatment is prolonged and slow and the results uncertain. The doctor can let them have a substantial analgesic and you must advise them about bed rest at home. It is all too easy simply to say lie flat on a hard mattress. The patient has to have someone to look after him (not everyone does). Some will not have a hard bed or a board to put under the mattress and may have to sleep on the carpet until the pain eases. Others think that bed rest means sitting up with a few pillows or just staying in bed for part of the day until they get fed up. You must advise about all such points to aid speedy recovery.

FACIOMAXILLARY INJURIES

Of prime importance is the fact that any of the following injuries can be accompanied by a head injury with all its added problems. In our high-speed world, it is now also common to see faciomaxillary injuries as just one part of generalized body trauma. Other injuries must be sought.

With several varieties of faciomaxillary injuries the airway can be in peril even if the patient has no accompanying head injury. If unconsciousness is added to the picture, the situation can be extremely urgent, requiring every ounce of skill you possess to keep the airway patent.

Special airway problems

Fractures of the mandible. With severe mandibular fractures the base of the tongue will have little support, falling backwards and blocking off the airway. Added to this is the fact that the fracture is commonly accompanied by a wound on the inside of the mouth, bleeding directly into the airway.

Care is threefold. Firstly, position the patient as you would with any unconscious patient (see Chapter 2), suck secretions and/or blood out of the mouth, using the laryngoscope if necessary. Secondly, support the jaw to some extent from behind the angle. Thirdly, if necessary, pull the tongue forwards using either dry gauze or tongue-holding forceps to get a firm grip. If all these measures fail urgent intubation will be required.

Middle-third fractures. The bones of the face can conveniently be divided into thirds (Fig. 122). If the middle third is fractured, it can be displaced backwards (dish face) (Fig. 123), therefore impinging to some extent on the airway. Apart from the usual airway care of positioning and suction, it may also be necessary to hold onto the mobile segment and pull it forwards with your fingers (Fig. 124).

Airway problems can also be caused by swallowed blood being vomited. Because of this danger, always try to position your patient so that the blood will trickle out of the nose or mouth. It is obvious that, if a patient's nose is blocked because of a blood clot or displacement of the middle third, the lips must be kept open or an airway inserted so that air can gain entry.

Extensive soft tissue injury

As you may have noticed if you have ever cut your face, it has an excellent blood supply. Bleeding, even from small wounds, can seem never-ending. With extensive soft tissue lacerations (as commonly seen with windscreen accidents), bleeding from the face can be very severe. Added to this the airway may be difficult to identify, let alone to keep clear.

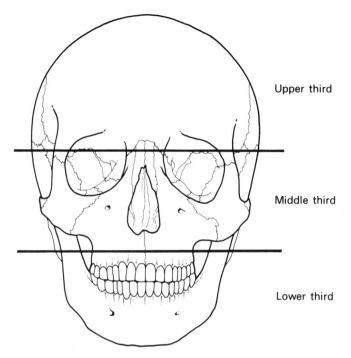

Fig. 122. *The bones of the face may be roughly divided into thirds.*

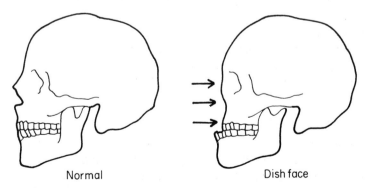

Fig. 123. *A 'dish' face caused by the bones of the middle third being pushed inwards. Common causes are kicks to the face and road traffic accidents. These outlines are taken from actual radiographs.*

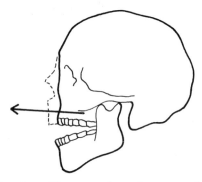

Fig. 124. *Pulling the middle segment forward may ease a blocked airway.*

General care of faciomaxillary injuries

The conscious patient can either sit up or lie down while being examined depending on how he feels. Before the doctor can see the injuries fully, excess blood will have to be removed from the face. Blood just inside and round the nostrils can be removed with moistened gauze wrapped round your finger, but deep clots should not be disturbed.

Epistaxis is rarely a problem by the time the patient arrives at hospital. I have never known a traumatic epistaxis to require packing on the unit. Indeed, if the nose continues to bleed your thoughts should drift to the possibility of a skull fracture with rhinorrhoea.

The eyelids should be opened on all patients, no matter how severe the surrounding swelling. It is a difficult task, but it is important to know if there is damage to the eye. Following road traffic accidents or pub violence, glass is occasionally driven into the eye and is easily missed in a patient with an altered level of consciousness.

Apart from the usual searches for swelling, grazes and bruises which may indicate a fracture, the doctor will also be on the alert for anaesthetic areas of skin by the cheek and the inside of the mouth. The margins of the orbits will be examined to discover any irregularity; ask about double vision and if the teeth 'meet' properly. These are pointers to fractures in the face.

Looking at the teeth is of special importance. With unconscious patients, just one tooth broken off and inhaled can cause tremendous trouble. If in doubt, a chest radiograph may be required to rule out the possibility of inhalation. For the patient who has an injury with a wound in the mouth, a mouthwash may be very pleasant. It will also help the doctor to see clearly inside.

When considering the shape of the nose following fractured nasal bones, what the patient says is of great importance. Look around you and see how many unusually shaped noses there are; this will help you to realize how difficult it is to judge the amount of displacement present following an injury. Another problem with fractures of the nasal bones is that the patient sometimes presents with the injury only on the next day and the swelling round the fracture site may be so severe that it is impossible for the doctor to judge if reduction is necessary. One final point about injuries to the nose: the doctor will always want to look inside the nostrils, probably using a Thudichum's speculum, to be sure that there is no haematoma in the nasal septum. If haematoma is present it will have to be drained to prevent it damaging the cartilage and worsening the deformity.

DISLOCATED JAW

Sometimes the jaw dislocates as an isolated incident but the condition can become recurrent. It often occurs as the patient yawns or shouts. The patient presents with mouth partly opened and unable to speak; saliva often drips from the corner of the mouth because swallowing is difficult. When communicating ensure that all your questions require simply a nod or a shake of the head.

Reduction of the dislocation is usually easy. The patient sits on a chair in front of the doctor, while the nurse stands behind or to one side to give reassurance. With both thumbs protected with folded gauze, the doctor presses downwards on the patient's back lower molars while the fingers ease under the angle of the jaw. After reduction the patient should be advised not to open the mouth excessively. Some suggest wearing a bandage for a while.

FURTHER READING

Heath, M.L. (1982) Deaths after i.v. regional anaesthesia. *British Medical Journal*, 285.
McRae, R. (1981) *Practical fracture treatment*, 1st edn. Edinburgh: Churchill Livingstone.

10 Lower limb and pelvic injuries

THE LOWER LIMB

The care and treatment of orthopaedic trauma is a field in which the nurse plays a very large part indeed. This fact alone makes it a particularly satisfying field in which to work. But, on the other side of the scale, there must be a far greater awareness of the complications which these treatments can produce. Another aspect of these injuries is that they will only rarely be the cause of a patient's death, so never allow their dramatic appearances and presentation to draw you away from the real emergencies: accompanying shock and head, chest and abdominal injuries. General care of the patient, for example, intravenous infusions, observation charts and taking of blood, will not be specially mentioned in each case described.

FRACTURES OF THE NECK OF FEMUR

The classical signs of shortening and external rotation are usually obvious pointers to the diagnosis. However, be wary of the patient having only hip pain. Some patients with impacted fractures can still walk!

The ideal treatment of femoral neck fractures, if the patient's general condition permits, is to operate as soon as possible. That will mean that shortly after arrival in the accident unit the patient will be going to theatre, and it will not, therefore, be worth while setting up temporary traction. After undressing the patient, support and analgesia are all that is practicable while on the accident and emergency unit. Methods to use include pillows, sandbags or a vacuum mattress (Fig. 125). Many patients with fractured femora are old ladies to whom hospital can be a very strange and frightening place and the thought of an operation completely alien. The patient may have long-thought herself too old for any

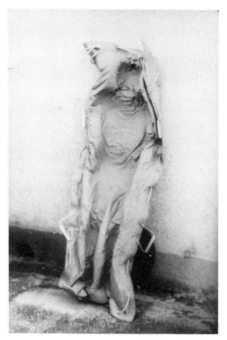

Fig. 125. *A vacuum mattress, here shown leaning up against a wall, to show how it maintains the shape of the body.*

surgery. Here then is a supreme example of how a nurse can settle her patient's mind. Take time to plug in the hearing aid if one is worn; explain that a neighbour is looking after the house, the family or the pets; find the phone number of the relative in Swansea! If the patient is confused try again and again to help her to understand where she is and what has happened. Last but not least, find out *why* she fell.

If the patient wants to pass urine while in the department a device such as the 'Feminal' made by Searle Medical may be far easier and less painful than a standard bedpan.

A word of warning: never allow an elderly person out of the department unless you have seen her walk successfully. If you do, some terrible mistake is bound to be made eventually. It is far too easy for an elderly person to be picked up after a fall, carried by the ambulance crew, wheeled into the accident and emergency unit, examined by the doctor, radiographed and wheeled out home again. In the whole process no one has seen whether she can walk. Seeing if an elderly patient can walk is a basic essential which is easily forgotten unless it is part of routine. If not, think to yourself: has anything been missed? where is the pain? were the x-rays complete?

This is a very good point at which to mention another question, apart from the purely technical aspects of the injury, which you must ask yourself before any patient leaves the department. It is especially relevant while talking here of elderly ladies with painful hips. The question is: 'Can the patient cope at home?' A fall and a bruise can convert a previously independent person to a cripple. The patient's background must be thoroughly looked into: find out if she lives on her own, what help she has, how she cooks, how often she sees people. I think that you will get quite a shock from some of the answers. Sometimes the general practitioner and community nurses will be able to step in to bridge the gap with the help of relations, social services department, Meals-on-Wheels and home helps. If not, the patient will have to be admitted.

On occasions I have had a secret prayer that a particular patient would have a fracture to ensure that he was admitted to hospital so that he could be cared for. Too often our medical colleagues look for fractures or medical conditions rather than at a patient who has suffered trauma and is unwell and temporarily unable to cope. To my mind until the community can adequately provide, the elderly should gain admission to hospital for supportive care and mobilization if injured, purely because often they cannot cope even when the injury is not something more tenable like a fracture.

FRACTURES OF THE FEMORAL SHAFT

Recognition of the fracture is the first essential. External rotation and shortening of the leg and a swollen thigh are the classical signs. Sometimes diagnosis is made even more obvious by gross angulation. In a baby unequal skin creases (Fig. 126) and telescoping also occurs.

After recognition get into the habit with all fractures of testing the movements, sensations and circulation to the limb concerned. From a legal point of view alone this is essential for you as the

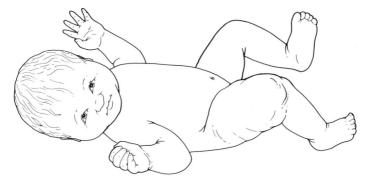

Fig. 126. *Unequal skin creases in the thigh may be caused by a fractured femur.*

nurse leader, so that you can be certain that you have not caused damage during any of your ministrations.

Initially with a fracture of the shaft of the femur the patient's blood volume must be replaced because the blood loss can be up to four pints.

We now have the problem of making the patient temporarily comfortable. The gigantic muscles contained in the thigh go into spasm with the slightest movement of the leg. The bones telescope into one another (Fig. 127). This causes excruciating pain, even in

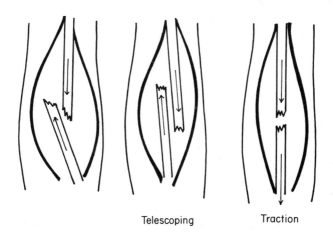

Telescoping   Traction

Fig. 127. *If a broken bone telescopes on itself, the result will be very painful. The result of traction, if firm and continuous, will be to free the patient of pain.*

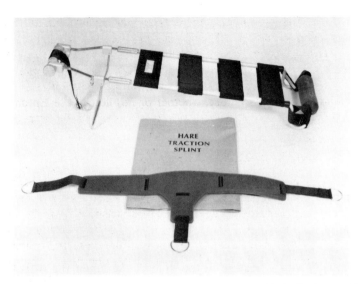

Fig. 128. *The Hare traction splint.* (**With kind permission of F.W. Equipment Co. Ltd**)

babies! The only way to counteract this effect is by applying continuous traction to the leg. I personally feel that it is kinder to apply a temporary Thomas splint or similar equivalent (Fig. 128) when the patient first arrives. (This is done with the aid of Entonox and/or intravenous pethidine.) It is very rare indeed that an adult will gain satisfactory pain relief from any other form of splintage. The continuous traction and immobilization of the leg will also help to slow down bleeding into the thigh. It is often found after radiography that this initial temporary splinting will be completely satisfactory. If this is not so, minor ward adjustments are occasionally all that are necessary. Of those that I have splinted myself over the years, roughly half were satisfactory at the first attempt, which I feel is a good record. The small degree of initial pain whilst the splint is applied is well balanced by firm efficient splinting after the first quarter of an hour. Once the splint is on, even if the fracture has not reduced itself sufficiently, the majority of the patient's pain will cease or be brought down to an easily bearable level. The wait of four to six hours while the stomach empties before a general anaesthetic will thus be less of an ordeal.

Most of the preceding comments concern young adults, but young children are a different matter. Because they do not understand much of what you are saying, every case must be judged with care on its merits. You must weigh up the amount of pain he is in, how long the wait for a general anaesthetic will be, the amount of displacement, whether or not he can use Entonox and whether or not gallows traction will be used on the ward.

Method of applying the Thomas splint

It seems very basic but the first essential of applying a Thomas splint is to give your patient an explanation of what is about to happen, why you are doing it and how the Entonox works. Be truthful and admit that there will be some pain. As long as he knows why you may cause a little pain some trust will remain. Skilful explanation often means the difference between a cooperative patient and a screaming uncooperative one. Measure the length of the patient's leg and add to this about 20 cm to give you the length of the splint. Next measure obliquely round the top of the thigh (Fig. 129) with the tape passing over the adductor

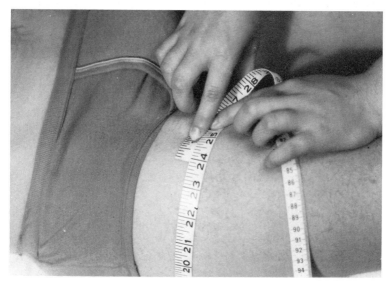

Fig. 129. *Measuring the size of the Thomas splint ring.*

tendon, ischial tuberosity and greater trochanter. Add to this a variable amount depending on the level of the fracture and experience, usually about 2–3 cm, to give you the internal diameter of the Thomas splint.

Apart from the splint itself all the remaining equipment necessary should be in sets ready for use.

Excessive dirt on the leg must be washed off and drying is of special importance if the strapping is to stick. I do not think shaving the leg is necessary unless it is very hairy. The leg has still not been moved, the part of the leg touching the bed is left until later. Lastly, gather an adequate number of experienced nurses around to help, delegate tasks and ensure that everyone understands exactly what will happen. It is important to realize that if the patient was having the fracture reduced and a splint applied under a general anaesthetic things would be different; it could all be done with a minimum of one nurse helping the doctor. However, in this present situation the patient is *only under a degree of analgesia* and all movements must be decisive, gentle and minimal if the patient is not to suffer. The Entonox is now started and must continue for two minutes if the patient is to gain full benefit.

One nurse stays at the head of the patient giving encouragement all the time. While the patient is inhaling, one side of the extension strapping can be applied (Fig. 130). Ensure that the malleoli are covered by foam or pads to prevent sores; some like the lateral aspect of the leg over the head of the fibula to be covered too, to prevent damage to the common peroneal nerve. I have never found Tinct. Benz. Co. to be necessary, although some people like it. While a nurse holds the foot and ankle and another supports the knee and fracture site (Fig. 131), traction is applied and the leg is gently and slowly brought so that the toes point to the ceiling. The traction on the leg is firm and continuous and is the major factor in preventing the patient from suffering. Before the days of Entonox this was still done with the utmost gentleness and can be done to young children with very little pain. The extension strapping is now brought round the other side of the leg and moulded to the contours. The strapping goes past the site of the fracture to the top of the thigh on either side. Bandages then hold the strapping in position and the splint is slid carefully over the leg into position ensuring that traction and support is continuous

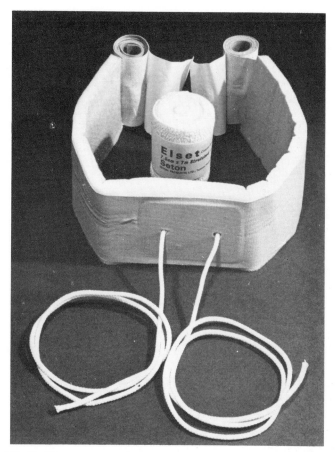

Fig. 130. *The Elset extension strapping kit.* (**With kind permission of Seton Products Ltd**)

throughout (Fig. 132). Three main slings and pads are then inserted (Fig. 133):

1. Under the proximal end of the distal fragment
2. Under the tibial condyles
3. Under the lower leg

Fill in with pads and slings elsewhere as needed.

Now that the patient's leg is resting on the splint the cords are passed round the splint (Fig. 134):

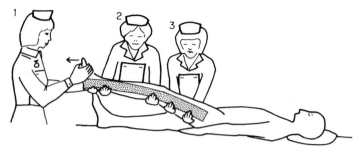

Fig. 131. *Nurse 1 holds the foot and ankle steady and applies continuous traction; Nurse 2 supports the knee and lower leg; Nurse 3 supports either side of the fracture.*

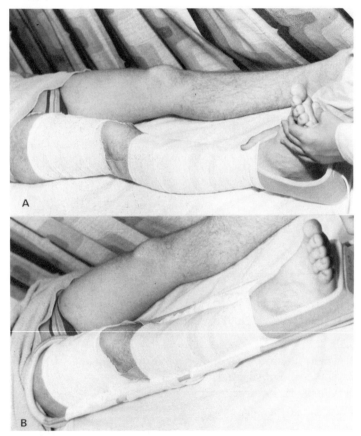

Fig. 132. A, *Bandages hold the extension strapping in position. Note that the knee is left free.* **B,** *The splint is gently manoeuvred over the leg and slings are then applied. Traction and support must be continuous through the procedure.*

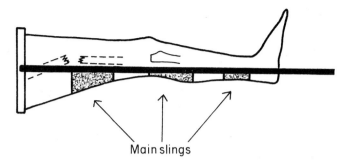

Fig. 133. *The position of the three main slings and pads of a Thomas splint.*

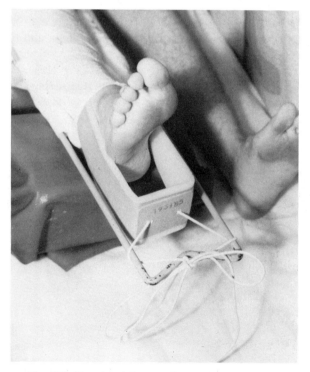

Fig. 134. *How the cords are tied on a Thomas splint.*

1. The medial cord goes:
     under bar
     over bar
     under end
2. The lateral cord goes:
     over bar
     under bar
     over end

Traction is applied to the leg a little more strongly while the cords are tied. Our job now completed, the end of the splint is placed on a support, the Entonox dispensed with and the movements, sensations and circulation to the toes tested to ensure that no harm has been done.

FRACTURES OF THE PATELLA AND UPPER END OF TIBIA

No matter what the design or extent of the fracture shown on the radiograph the main findings in fractures of patella and tibia are the same: pain and tenderness over the patella or tibia and in most cases a haemarthrosis (blood in the joint) (Fig. 135). A small haemarthrosis can just be left, but if of any reasonable size it will require aspiration, once again in a theatre to avoid infection.

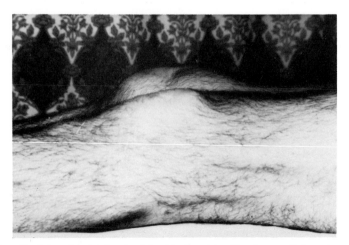

Fig. 135. *A huge haemarthrosis of the right knee joint. Note how easily it can be seen when compared with the good knee.*

Fractures which will require operation are temporarily supported with wool, crêpe and a splint extending down the back of the leg. However, if conservative treatment is to be followed one of two treatments will be given:

1. A Robert Jones bandage plus a back splint and crutches.
2. A firm wool and crêpe bandage with a plaster cylinder applied over the top. Once again the patient will require crutches.

If a back splint is being applied, ensure that it does not dig in at the top or slide down and rub on the Achilles tendon every time the patient moves (Fig. 136). Warn the patient that slight swelling of the foot may occur because of the firmness of the bandages. Show how the leg can be kept well elevated on a stool when not walking about, presuming of course that the condition is mild enough for the patient to go home. With all these injuries ensure that movements, sensations and circulation to the limb are satisfactory; this cannot be stressed too much.

Before I finish with the knee completely I wish to make a brief mention about the ligaments and what is said applies to many other parts of the body. Just because a radiograph shows that nothing is fractured, that does not necessarily mean that everything is all right. An inexperienced casualty officer may have missed something else. The medial, lateral and cruciate ligaments, plus the extensor mechanism, must all be examined to ensure that they are not torn. This is of especial importance when you are faced with a patient who has been radiographed but nothing found and who has then been discharged, yet is still in intense pain (out of all proportion to a mild injury) and cannot walk. Always be guided by the patient's appearance, not the radiograph, and look deeper into the matter.

DISLOCATION OF THE KNEE

I have seen a few knee dislocations; it is very rare and very serious. Test the movements, sensations and circulation to the toes immediately on admission. There is a great danger of damage to the popliteal vessels and nerves. Immobilize the limb in a position which is both comfortable for the patient and affords the leg a good blood supply. Senior orthopaedic assistance will be needed.

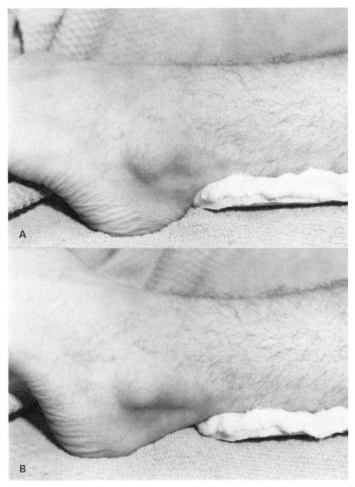

Fig. 136. *When applying a back splint to the leg, ensure that the skin over the Achilles tendon does not dig in when the foot is moved,* **A.** *The correct position is shown in* **B.**

DISLOCATION OF THE PATELLA

In comparison to dislocation of the knee, dislocation of the patella is quite common and is not associated with damage to any vessels or nerves. The patella usually dislocates laterally and the injury tends to recur. Classically the patient (a youngster) arrives in great discomfort, with the knee bent to about 45°. The deformity is obvious, with the patella 'flipped' over to one side. This dislocation reduces so easily that even a bumpy ambulance ride can occasionally do the trick. The nurse's first job is to relax the anxious patient and gain his confidence. The leg will then be very gently straightened while reassuring the patient. The doctor will press gently on the lateral side of the patella, pushing it inwards. I have never known a patient require a general anaesthetic for this procedure and even analgesia is required only rarely. After reduction the knee is supported with a Robert Jones bandage and the patient is given a stick for a day or two.

FRACTURES OF THE TIBIA AND FIBULA

A fracture of the tibia and fibula is a very common injury, especially on Saturday afternoon when the footballers start coming in ! First ask the patient to tell you exactly where the pain is. If the patient is a footballer, undo all the football boot laces or cut through them as the patient wishes. Ask a colleague to hold the ankle firmly while you gently ease off the boot (Fig. 137). Next comes the sock; footballers have a habit of tying string or laces

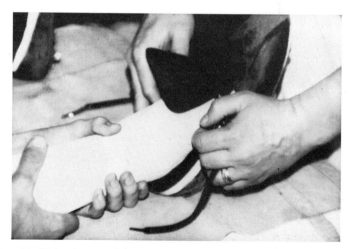

Fig. 137. *With a fracture of the leg the lower part of the limb is held firmly while the boot is gently eased off.*

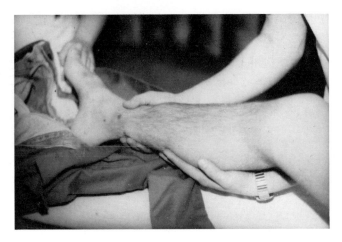

Fig. 138. *Holding a fractured leg firmly yet gently.*

round the tops of their socks and then folding the top over, so ensure that you do not forget to cut this. Slide the sock down gently while the leg is still being held (Fig. 138). If this causes pain ask the patient if you can cut it off.

If your patient is not a footballer and has trousers which need removing (Fig. 139) these must first be eased down to the

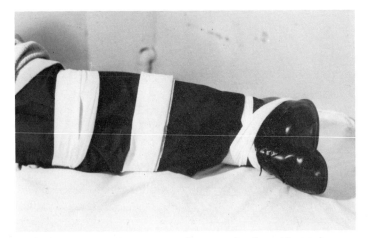

Fig. 139. *How a fractured leg is commonly presented to the accident and emergency staff. It requires skill and patience to undress and splint such cases.*

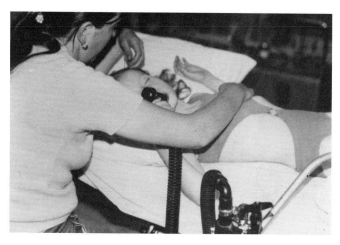

Fig. 140. *This little girl waited four hours before her fracture could be reduced. She is quite happy here despite the severe displacement of bones because she has her Mum and the Entonox.*

mid-thigh region while the leg is well supported. Entonox may be necessary, depending on your patient and the type of fracture (Fig. 140). Next the good knee is bent and the leg eased out. It may then take two or three nurses to remove the trousers painlessly from the injured limb while keeping the fracture steady.

Before anything else is done the movements, sensations and circulation to the limb must be tested.

Immobilization is next. There are several methods, each of which has its advantages. The inflatable splint and 'box' splint are about the most common methods in current use with the ambulance service (Fig. 141). The inflatable splint can be used to great benefit with compound fractures, where the pressure helps to stop bleeding, and in my many years of trauma experience I have yet to see one seriously interfere with the circulation to the limb. I have also found it unnecessary to deflate it at intervals. Entonox is once again sometimes required for the application of the splint, but there are many instances where, with enough helpers and a thorough explanation to the patient, it can be applied without. Most fractures from the knee downwards can be effectively immobilized with a full leg splint. Ensure that the design is such that the zip goes up to the toes, otherwise it will be difficult to

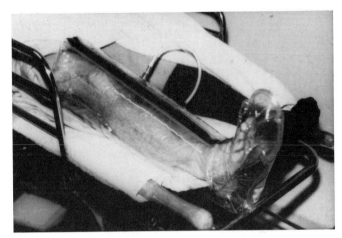

A

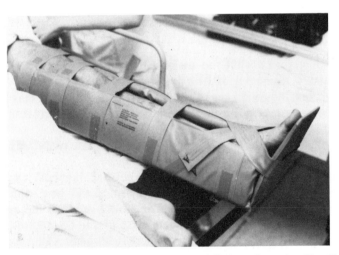

B

Fig. 141. A, *A footballer with a fractured tibia and fibula made comfortable with an inflatable splint.* **B,** *The use of a 'box' splint for a fractured lower leg.*

apply. Lastly, let your patient be your guide; if after all your trouble it hurts even more (which sometimes happens), take it off and try an alternative.

Vac-Pac splints are a useful alternative which I feel will find a great use in accident and emergency departments (Fig. 142).

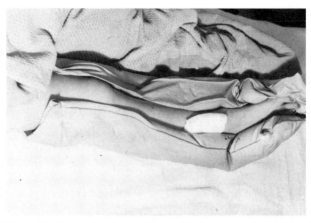

Fig. 142. *A Vac-Pac splint keeps the leg of the unconscious patient firmly immobilized and allows ample view of the patient's wound.*

These contain granules which bind firmly together when the air is sucked out of the PVC cover. The splint then attains boardlike rigidity and will hold a fractured limb in any position. Lastly, remember that sandbags and/or pillows still have a large part to play and give great relief.

Treatment

Whole books have been written on the treatment of these fractures alone. Briefly, I want to state the following guidelines. A compound fracture with anything more than a tiny puncture wound will require exploration, toilet and suture in a theatre. All patients with compound fractures should be admitted. A closed fracture of the shaft will probably have to be reduced under a general anaesthetic and a long leg plaster of Paris applied. Comparatively trivial fractures, such as undisplaced cracks, will require only analgesia for the application of plaster of Paris.

The decision as to whether the patient goes home or not depends on several factors:

1. How serious a fracture is it?
2. Is it reduced satisfactorily?
3. How much pain is the patient in?
4. What is the circulation like?

5. What are the home conditions like?
6. Is the patient steady with the crutches?

Fractures of the lower end of the tibia and fibula

With these fractures the treatment varies but a cold pack laid across the ankle can ease swelling considerably while the patient is awaiting x-ray (Fig. 143). If the fracture is severe, the care will be the same as for a shaft injury, that is reduction and long leg plaster of Paris. If the injury is a minor fracture of the lateral malleolus, the treatment varies enormously from hospital to hospital. Some examples are below-knee plaster, wool and crêpe or Elastoplast (Fig. 144). With all the above treatments the patient will be non-weight-bearing at first and will require crutches to help mobility. The nurse has a duty to teach the patient how to use these correctly, not merely to hand them over. The more elderly and frail patients may require a Zimmer walking aid instead.

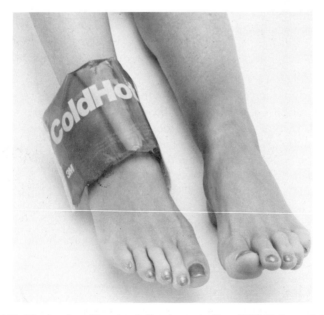

Fig. 143. *The use of a cold pack to help to lessen swelling.* (**With kind permission of 3M UK Ltd**)

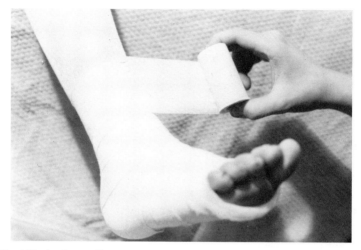

Fig. 144. *Applying adhesive elastic strapping holding on to the edges of the spool.*

FRACTURES OF THE FOOT

I will mention two types of fracture here: firstly, fracture of the base of the fifth metatarsal which is quite a common injury, and secondly, fractures of the heel bone (calcaneum) which are seen less commonly.

Fractured base of the fifth metatarsal

Fractures of the fifth metatarsal base are caused by an inversion strain applied to the foot (that is the sole of the foot is forced inwards). This occurs, for instance, when a step is missed coming down stairs or the foot wrenched on uneven ground. Initial care consists of support by one of the methods listed under ankle sprains plus non-weight-bearing with crutches. Mild analgesics may be required but pain should not be severe once the fracture is supported.

Fractures of the calcaneum

The classical way of fracturing the calcaneum is to land heavily on the heel. Although operation is rarely required, the majority of

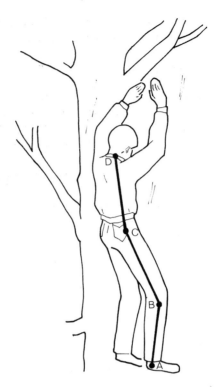

Fig. 145. *If a falling person lands on his heels, the shock waves travel up the body. Injuries distant from the site of impact may occur, commonly involving the tibia, the lumbar vertebrae and the base of the skull.*

patients are fairly comfortable with wool and crêpe from toes to knee plus elevation. A strong drug such as pethidine or pentazocine may be required for the pain, which may be severe.

The seriousness of these fractures lies in the possibility of simultaneous injury to other parts of the body which may easily be missed unless you are 'on your toes'. Fig. 145 shows how the shock wave of landing on your heels can travel. Always look for:

1. Fractures of the other heel (common)
2. Fractures of the tibiae
3. Compression fractures of the lumbar vertebrae (common)
4. Fractures of the base of the skull

This fracture is the ideal example of the importance of always asking your patient 'how the accident occurred'.

FRACTURES OF THE TOES

Toe fractures are very common injuries especially in men working in industry. The usual story is that something has fallen on the foot and the patient was not wearing shoes with safety linings. The fractures usually involve the terminal phalanges and are frequently compound or associated with a collection of blood under the toe-nail (subungual haematoma). Blisters filled with blood are also frequently seen.

If the fracture is closed, place cotton wool between the toes to prevent intertrigo and strap the injured toe to its companion; reduction is rarely necessary. An alternative is to use Tubifoam (Fig. 146).

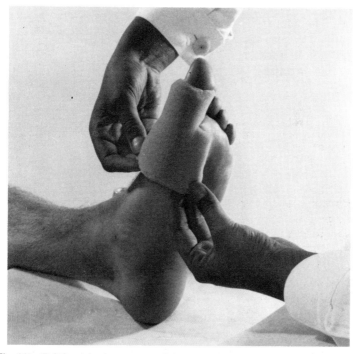

Fig. 146. *Tubifoam used to protect a fractured toe.* (**With kind permission of Seton Products Ltd**)

Although it sounds very obvious, warn the patient against accidental stubbing of the toe; it is very easy and will cause excruciating pain. Advise cutting the end out of an old slipper to ease pressure. The patient will have to walk on a part of the foot that does not hurt and will perhaps require crutches or a stick depending on how severe the injury is. Placing a pad of felt on the sole of the foot under the metatarsal heads can help to keep weight off the toes and is also worth a try (Fig. 147).

MENISCUS INJURIES

The menisci sit on top of the tibial plateau as shown in Fig. 148. They deepen and strengthen the knee joint. They are most commonly injured in football players when the foot is fixed in the ground and the player twists around with all the weight on a slightly flexed knee. Because of its firm attachments the medial (inside) meniscus is torn more frequently than the lateral (outside). The patient will present with a painful knee; often he will mention previous episodes and may even be listed for operation. There will be tenderness over the affected cartilage and the joint may have a varying degree of effusion (collection of fluid in the joint).

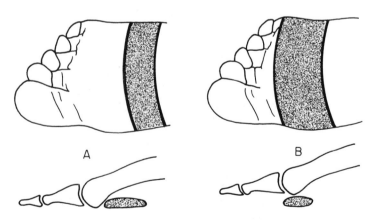

Fig. 147. *Some people treat fractures of the toes with pads under the foot. Position* **A**, *the standard position for a metatarsal pad, will give little relief. Position* **B** *eases the pain as the toes will not be used much during walking.*

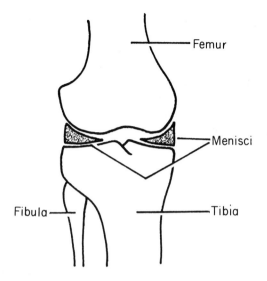

Fig. 148. *The position of the menisci on top of the tibial plateau.*

One final point: the patient may be unable to straighten the knee joint completely (locking); bending it is possible. This is often caused by the cartilage being trapped between the articular surfaces.

Most of your patients with meniscus injuries will require only a Robert Jones bandage with crutches, analgesics and an appointment for the next orthopaedic clinic.

If knee straightening is considerably restricted a general anaesthetic may be necessary so that the joint can be manipulated and a back splint applied. Minor degrees of locking, however, may be caused by muscle spasm which will gradually ease as the pain subsides.

The Robert Jones bandage

Originally a Robert Jones bandage was a layer of cotton wool from just above the ankle to the top of the leg, covered by a firm domette bandage. The whole process was then repeated twice more, so that you finished up with three layers of wool and three layers of domette. Most hospitals still use the name Robert Jones, but modify the layers for accident and emergency work. A typical example would be to use only two instead of three layers and crêpe instead of domette. The bandage gives very firm support indeed, but allows a few degrees of movement. It is ideally suited to limiting and helping to disperse an effusion or haemarthrosis in the knee joint.

Any large effusion into the joint will require aspiration. This procedure must be done under fully sterile conditions in a theatre. Although it seems a simple enough procedure, the knee joint itself is entered and the possibility of bacteria entering and the patient developing a septic arthritis just does not bear thinking about.

THE SPRAINED ANKLE

The sprained ankle can be termed the 'bread and butter' of the accident and emergency department. It is often as painful and as crippling as a fracture, but many nurses mistakenly believe that, just because nothing is broken, it is a trivial injury. It can vary from its simplest form, where it produces little more than a slight limp, to a very severe injury which will have your patient off work for many weeks and unable to put the foot to the ground.

Treatments are many and vary both with the severity of the injury and with the particular likes of the doctor in question. The general routine is as follows:

1. If the discomfort is trivial, allow weight-bearing. If moder-ate, give the patient a stick. If severe, give the patient crutches.
2. Give firm support with, for example, a crêpe bandage, wool and crêpe, or elastic adhesive strapping, double Tubigrip, crêpe on Tubigrip or plaster of Paris (below-knee).
3. Rest the joint at first and elevate the leg when not in use. Encourage movements of the toes.
4. As soon as the acute pain eases, start ankle movements and gradually mobilize.

The majority of your patients will be over the worst of the injury in about 10 days, but may still require support such as one layer of Tubigrip and need encouragement to exercise actively.

In the more severe forms, where the lateral ligament of the

ankle has been badly damaged, the plaster of Paris or strapping may have to be worn for three weeks or more.

Points about applying the support

The crêpe bandage. A 10 cm (4 in) crêpe bandage is ideal for this task in the average adult, although you will find that to give firm support the bandage may not be long enough and a second one may have to be started. It should extend from the base of the toes to just below the knee in practically all patients. Do not adhere to the 'pretty' patterns shown in many books; these were thought of many years ago when patients were immobile for weeks on end and will just not stand up to the pressures of today's patient. Without advising a regular pattern, all I can say about application is that you should have several even thicknesses of crêpe round each part, firmly applied so that it will give good support. Ensure that it moulds neatly to the contours of the leg without creases. Lastly, and this applies to most treatments described in this chapter and Chapter 9, watch a skilled accident and emergency sister show you how, first of all, so that you start off on the right track. Unlike those on the wards, your patient is soon gone and it is then too late to rectify mistakes, so the task must be done correctly first time.

Elastic adhesive strapping. Slightly different rules apply with elastic adhesive strapping. Always ask if your patient has an allergy to plaster first. Apply a layer of tube gauze to the limb so that the plaster does not stick to the patient's hairs. Then apply the strapping as shown in Fig. 144, holding the ends of the spool only and taking care not to press the layers together. Cover the leg as evenly as possible; excessive layers in just part of the leg will cause constriction, pain and swelling. Be even more careful than with crêpe not to get any creases. You will find that a 7.5 cm (3in) roll is far easier to apply than the 10 cm (4in), which often has to be heaved to make it move at all. One and a half of the 7.5 cm (3 in) bandages should be satisfactory for an adult, toes to knee.

Tubigrip. Tubigrip doubled over initially gives good firm support for the injury and later can be altered to a single layer as swelling subsides. A single layer of 10 cm (4 in) crêpe on top is also very effective indeed in the early stages and is far less bulky than crêpe over wool, enabling the patient to wear a shoe.

Footwear

If, even with the help of a shoehorn, the shoe will still not fit, ask your patient to walk on the uppers (Fig. 149). The shoe can be

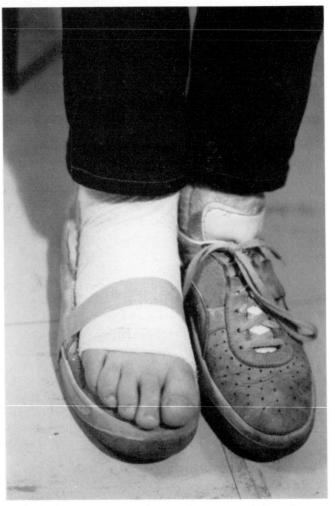

Fig. 149. *If the patient's shoe will not fit he can walk temporarily on the upper with the shoe attached to his foot by strapping. Once he is at home he can use the same principle with a slipper and elastic bands.*

held in place temporarily with strapping, as shown, until the patient fixes something better at home. While on the subject of footwear, mention should also be made of some of the very unstable styles which are very common in the shops. Although it is almost impossible to persuade some young girls to change their shoe styles, a temporary change to a flatter sole should be strongly hinted at, at least until the ankle has a chance to settle down again.

THE PELVIS

FRACTURES OF THE PELVIS

Recognition of pelvic fracture is not always as straight-forward as you would think. Although diagnosis is fairly easy after a road traffic accident when the patient is in acute pain, if the patient is unconscious a routine radiograph of the pelvis will have to be taken so that a fracture is never missed. Also, with an elderly patient complaining of pain in the hip, it is very easy for the femur to be scrutinized and the pelvis forgotten.

It is important to be aware of the enormous size of the pelvic girdle and the amount of blood that can be lost inside (three units easily and occasionally many more).

Look at the external urethral meatus to see if there is any blood; this plus inability to pass urine points strongly towards a ruptured urethra. In this instance on no account pass a catheter until senior surgical advice has been sought, in case more damage is done. Contusion of the bladder is very common, the patient passing blood-stained urine. Rupture of the bladder occurs far less frequently; the patient will not be able to micturate or may pass with difficulty only minute amounts of heavily blood-stained urine. If this occurs coax the patient not to try to pass urine any more.

Lastly, I would like to give a brief mention to a complication which can rapidly exsanguinate the patient. This is damage to one of the major blood vessels, for example the internal iliac artery. Haemorrhage will be torrential and progressive; early operation is essential.

Actual positive treatment for the fracture itself cannot start properly until the patient arrives on the ward and can be attached to traction apparatus. However, by your general gentleness in undressing the patient and by moving any seriously ill patient as little as possible, you can considerably ease suffering and bleeding.

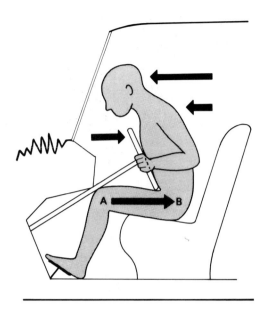

Fig. 150. *A common cause of posterior dislocation of the hip is banging the knees against the dashboard in a car accident,* **A**, *creating a force which pushes the femora backwards,* **B**.

DISLOCATION OF THE HIP

Hip dislocation occurs fairly frequently. The usual cause of the more common posterior dislocation is shown in Fig. 150. It is commonly associated with grazes or fractures round the knee. The position of the patient's leg is fairly typical and should help you to recognize the injury at once (Fig. 151). The pain of these large dislocations is so sickening that the patients may forget to tell you of other lesser injuries or the ever-important abdominal pain associated with intra-abdominal trauma. Be on your guard. Never think of your patient as having a dislocated hip, but rather as someone whose body has been subjected to terrific forces and will need careful observation to ensure that nothing else is damaged and an i.v. cannula. Your patient will find a great deal of difficulty in discovering a comfortable position and will require great patience and tact. Several pillows and foam may be necessary, even after analgesics. Your next job as a nurse is to check once again the movements, sensations and circulation to the limb.

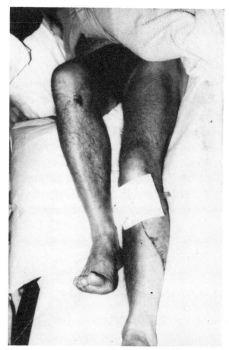

Fig. 151. *A posterior dislocation of the hip. Note how the affected leg is flexed and internally rotated; both knees have grazes where they hit the dashboard.*

Treatment is reduction of the joint under a general anaesthetic. One major difference is that the surgeon may want to reduce the dislocation with the patient on the floor. Be prepared for this and put poles ready in the canvas, and provide anaesthetic tubing of adequate length.

FURTHER READING

McRae, R. (1981) *Practical fracture treatment*, 1st edn. London: Churchill Livingstone.

11 Acute poisoning

Acute poisoning is an unpleasant and ever-increasing section of our work. It takes up a great deal of our time and requires much skill and understanding. Treatment, especially of the unconscious patient, is fraught with dangers. Despite all our efforts, a substantial number of our patients will either succeed in their original aim or, when exposed to the pressures of the outside world, will 'try, try and try again'. With adults accidental poisoning is a rarity.

For the purpose of this book, I will divide the patients roughly into three groups: the conscious adult, the conscious child and the unconscious patient. Finally, I will finish with a list of the common poisons and their treatment. With all cases 'treat what you find'. It is rare for a specific antidote to exist.

THE CONSCIOUS ADULT

Acute poisoning in a conscious adult is a difficult aspect of accident and emergency nursing, mainly because you are often faced with someone who does not appear to want to be helped. Note that I said 'appear'. These patients are often severely troubled and may be desperately in need of support. Sadly, in an accident and emergency environment, we do not have enough time at our disposal to build any sort of relationship. Indeed, to a large extent excessive sympathy shown to such patients on arrival is not wise. An understanding but firm approach is the best throughout the patient's stay.

History

To start with, it is important that a full history is obtained from the patient, any relations, friends, passers-by or the ambulance men. It is only with this thorough history, plus tablet or chemical containers and an examination, that a correct diagnosis can be made by the doctor. In all cases ask about the following:

1. The exact name of the drug or substance
2. The strength of the drug

  3. The number of tablets taken
  4. When the substance was taken
  5. Was any alcohol taken with the drug?
  6. Why was the drug taken?
  7. Has the patient vomited; if so, what did the vomitus contain?
  8. Does the patient have any serious illnesses?
  9. Are any children left at home? Are they being cared for? Are they safe?
  10. Who is the next of kin?

General care

Ensure that the patients are not left alone to harm themselves further. Confiscate any remaining tablets. I have known patients to have tablets hidden in property and take more when no one was around. Try to be an understanding listener and gain the patient's confidence. If some basics of a relationship can be achieved, sometimes even an aggressive patient can be subdued by a particular nurse who has befriended him. In most instances the stomach will have to be emptied either by giving an emetic or a stomach washout. The method will depend on the substance taken and local procedures. If you are ever in doubt about the need for an emetic or washout, remember the fact that a patient who really wanted to kill himself would lie to you about the number of tablets and the time at which they were taken!

Emetic

With an adult patient 30–45 ml ipecacuanha followed by a glass of water will usually work.

The stomach washout

Firstly, never perform a stomach washout until the patient has been examined and certified as fit by the casualty officer; an 'over-the-phone message' is not good enough and will eventually lead to disaster.

  Prepare all the equipment away from the patient's sight. Nothing is more likely to make the patient agitated and induce him to refuse the tube than staring at it lying on a nearby trolley (Fig. 152).

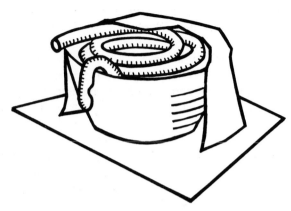

Fig. 152. *If you saw this coming towards you, would you wait to see what it was for? Always keep equipment like this covered or out of sight.*

Equipment. You will require the following:

Powerful suction
Equipment for artificial ventilation
Stomach tube
Tubing and connection (if the stomach tube is the short type)
Funnel
Lubricant
Two large jugs of water at approximately body temperature
Bucket
Large bowl
Some form of gag
Paper towels
Laboratory specimen container

The size and type of tube are quite important. I have frequently heard nurses say 'it will be kinder to use a narrow tube'. In fact, nothing could be further from the truth. A wide-bore stomach tube, size 35 FG, is ideal for the majority of adults. Only with such a wide bore can large particles of food and whole tablets come through. Small tubes block easily. Nothing is worse than passing a small tube, then having to remove it and pass another because it has become blocked. I hardly ever use any other lubricant on the tube except plain water. However, if you prefer, use a little KY jelly or liquid paraffin. Some use a Ferguson gag to hold the jaws open, but I feel this is being a little severe. In most instances, a padded spatula or its equivalent is all that is necessary.

Procedure. Explain to the patient what is to happen, but avoid a vivid description as it may frighten the patient into refusing. Remember that to attempt a washout on an unwilling patient is a criminal assault and could lead you into a very tricky legal situation. If the patient refuses and the washout is essential, a psychiatrist will have to be called. Only if he agrees that the patient is unstable and places the patient in the care of the hospital can you proceed legally. Thankfully, however, this situation is very rare. With tact most patients will eventually agree to treatment, even though they will not exactly help you to get the tube down!

Positioning. A head-down tilt on an accident trolley is the best position, although in extreme cases (i.e. orthopnoeic patients) the washout can be done with the patient sitting up. The patient lies on the right side. The cot sides are raised, the pillow removed and the canvas rolled down to the shoulders. Remove any false teeth, placing them safely in a special, labelled container so they are not lost or forgotten. Position all your equipment and get a nurse to hold the patient's wrists securely. I make a point of having the tube resting in the bowl under the trolley. This is well out of the sight of the patient and what he cannot see will not cause any fear.

Passing the tube. Ask the patient to open the mouth. Place a gag in the corner between the teeth to prevent the jaws being closed. Now introduce the tube gently over the tongue towards the back of the throat. Ask the patient to swallow and at the same time introduce the tube further. You will feel it 'give' as it starts its journey down the oesophagus. Ask the patient to continue swallowing and push it down fairly quickly (about another 30 cm) into the stomach. As soon as it touches the back of the throat your patient will reflexly try to bring up the hands and drag it out; this is why another nurse must hold the patient's wrists firmly before you start. Passing the tube should only require the pressure of two fingers (Fig. 153). It is difficult, but not impossible, to intubate the larynx with the tube, but fairly frequently the tube is unable to pass the back of the tongue because of the patient's involuntary

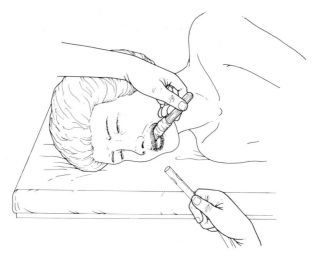

Fig. 153. *Passing the stomach tube. Firm but gentle pressure is required.*

resistance. At any time during the passage of the tube, and afterwards, be on the alert for struggling and jerky head movements which can easily force the tube out again. If you have your left hand and forearm holding the head as shown in Fig. 153, this problem will be minimized. Once the patient drags or jerks the tube out he will be far less willing to have it put back.

Some difficulties. The problem of a mouth which will not open occasionally arises. Here, tact and superhuman patience are necessary. In many instances though, the situation would not have occurred if the patient had not been allowed a glimpse of the tube before it was passed or if the operator had put the gag in firmly the first time and held on correctly. The passing of a stomach tube on a frightened patient is not a job for a 'ditherer'.

Cold polythene disposable tubes tend to be hard and can injure the patient as they are passed. To avoid this place them in warm water until they are supple. Alternatively, use the standard red rubber tube, which even when cold is soft and only rarely injures the mucosa. Doubling up of the tube sometimes occurs and should be borne in mind if no flow results after a difficult passage.

Continued retching can be caused by movement of the tube irritating the pharynx. It can be eased if the tube is held to the

corner of the mouth and not allowed to hang free. If excessive
retching continues, speak authoritatively and reassuringly to the
patient. Coax him to stop and stress that he will not choke and is in
no danger. This simple reassurance, which may have to be
continued, can work miracles.

When the tube is in the stomach. Soon after the tube is in the
stomach, gastric contents will start to run out. There is no need to
test this with litmus paper; it must be from the stomach. With
some individuals gas is expelled under force through the gastric
tube; this is caused by the stomach contracting forcibly. Although
the noise can seem like breath sounds there is no need to worry so
long as your patient is 'pink' and not in any respiratory distress.
Keep the first concentrated fluid which runs out as a specimen.
When this initial flow has ceased, pour in the first 100 ml or so of
water. Then turn the funnel down over the bucket and let it
syphon out. Continue to pour about 250–500 ml in at a time and
then avert the funnel until the water runs clear. It can take a long
time!

More difficulties. If fluid will not run in, the cause in most cases
will be blockage of the tube lumen by debris (for instance, a hunk
of food or large tablet), kinking or the patient biting (Fig. 154).
Very occasionally it can be because of the tube 'doubling up'
inside the oesophagus. To clear a blocked tube, first try raising the
funnel as high as possible and looking inside the mouth for biting
or kinking (Fig. 154F, G). If this does not work, kink the tube with
your fingers and squeeze a section on the tubing nearer the patient
(Fig. 155), then immediately open up the tube again. This has the
effect of pumping water down the tube, which may unblock it. If
unsuccessful, remove the tube, clear it and then insert it again.
Always ensure that you return a quantity of fluid similar to that
which you have put in. If not, the tube may have a piece of food in
it flapping about like a valve, thus allowing fluid to flow mainly in
one direction (Fig. 154C, D). If you are not wary of this, massive
vomiting can occur round the tube, which is unpleasant and
dangerous for the patient, and messy for you. Other causes of no
fluid return are:

1. Tube not in the stomach

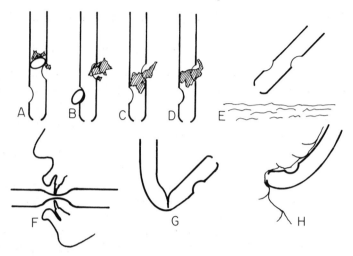

Fig. 154. *Stomach tube problems.* **A**, **B** *The tube may be blocked by food or tablets.* **C**, **D**, *Debris in the tube may act as a valve, allowing water into the stomach but not out.* **E**, *The tube may not be far enough in.* **F**, *The patient may bite the tube.* **G**, *kinking of the tube may occur in the mouth, oesophagus or stomach.* **H**, *The tube may rest against the stomach wall so that flow is prevented.*

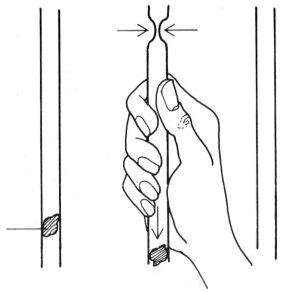

Fig. 155. *A simple method of clearing a blocked stomach tube.*

2. End of the tube blocked by the wall of stomach or food (Fig. 154H)
3. End of tube away from stomach contents (Fig. 154E)

Throughout the washout, intermittent suction will be necessary in most cases. This must be done in short spells so as not to 'take the patient's breath away'. Do not be alarmed by suction of blood; this will usually be caused by minor trauma to the pharynx when the tube is passed and it soon ceases.

When the washout fluid is clear, allow all contents to drain away. Then kink the tube so that no fluid escapes and withdraw it fairly quickly. Very rarely, especially with very nervous patients, the tube cannot be withdrawn. If this occurs, continue with gentle continuous traction to the tube along with plenty of reassurance. Eventually, over about ten minutes, the patient's muscle spasm will slowly relax and the tube will 'inch' its way out to everyone's relief.

Finally clean the patient up to make him feel comfortable.

CONSCIOUS CHILDREN

With poisoning in children we obviously have a completely different picture: classically, a happy smiling toddler, wondering what all the fuss is about, accompanied by an anxious, worried, crying mother.

Treatment is aimed at:

1. Finding out the precise details of the poison (Fig. 156)
2. Settling the parents down and reassuring them
3. Emptying the child's stomach

The emptying of the stomach can be done either by stomach washout as with an adult or, more commonly, by giving 15 ml of ipecacuanha orally, followed by a glass of water which can be flavoured with orange or other juice, if available. After a wait of about 20 minutes the child almost always vomits a few times. If not, the dose is repeated and more water is given. I have never known a second dose not to work. Always send a specimen of the vomit to the laboratory.

If a stomach washout is required, it is obvious that a small size tube will be required. However, never make it too small out of 'kindness'. A broad guide is that a toddler can usually cope with a

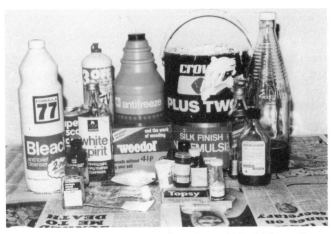

Fig. 156. *Some of the amazing range of products which children will eat. This collection was made over only one month.*

28FG tube. With washouts in children, make 101 per cent sure that they do not catch sight of any of the equipment before you start; it will terrify them. Even when you are about to pass the tube, hold it down underneath the trolley so that it cannot be seen. Before the procedure starts have the child securely wrapped up in a small blanket. This gives a feeling of security and makes him far more manageable. Talk to the child, stroke the head and reassure constantly throughout the ordeal. I do not usually ask parents to stay, but if they specifically ask I allow it gladly because any comfort the child can get is useful.

While mentioning the parents: remember to explain why an anaesthetic cannot be given, otherwise misunderstandings can occur and they may think of the nurses as being cruel.

The amount of fluid poured into the stomach each time will vary considerably with the child's size. If too much is put in, unnecessary vomiting will occur, so be on the alert for this.

If you are in any way suspicious about the way the poisoning occurred, for instance an outright case of neglect or deliberate poisoning:

1. Refer to senior medical staff, who may wish to keep the child in hospital.

2. Inform the social services department and the health visitors of your suspicions.

THE UNCONSCIOUS PATIENT

The overriding consideration in the unconscious patient is the airway. The treatment of this has already been explained in detail in Chapter 2. However, brief mention must be made here of some specific points.

1. Unconsciousness varies in its degrees. Some patients will require intubation with a cuffed endotracheal tube prior to stomach washout. In others, unconsciousness may be so light that a tube will not be tolerated. The airway, however, is in far more danger than with the fully conscious. A washout here is a perilous undertaking, carrying a low but significant mortality.
2. The level of consciousness will often not remain static. As more of the drug is absorbed, the deeper the unconsciousness becomes and therefore the more perilous the washout.
3. Any situation which involves an unconscious patient and several litres of water is bound to be dangerous.

If at all in doubt about whether the patient can cope with an endotracheal tube, insist on an anaesthetist being called to decide. If an intravenous infusion is to be set up, have it done after the washout, if possible, not before, as struggling often rips out the tube.

DRUG ADDICTION PROBLEMS

Most accident and emergency departments throughout Great Britain see an occasional drug addict. This is often someone who tries to obtain drugs by faking illness, for example renal colic or chest pain, in the hope that pethidine or heroin will be given. To avert this situation, all patients must be examined thoroughly and every accident and emergency specialist nurse should make a point of looking for injection marks or thrombosed veins which may give a hint and lead to the correct diagnosis. To this end it is also important to keep an up-to-date list of such people and pass information on to other hospitals.

The major drug problem is, however, seen mainly by certain of the inner London hospitals, or perhaps in hospitals in the centres of other big cities, and is rather different. Here the picture is a tragic one of districts with known high concentrations of addicts. Addiction has become a way of life for them and they need regular injection to get any sort of relief or meaning from life. Frequently the patients are found in varying degrees of 'collapse', hanging round the streets or slumped in a corner. An ambulance is called by a passer-by and the patient ends up in the accident and emergency department. Little of lasting effect can be done for them in the accident and emergency department. All have to be examined to ensure that drugs are the cause of the state. Infected intravenous injection marks may be found in the elbows, forearms, hands and even fingers caused by poor technique and re-use of needles and syringes. Most are left to 'sleep it off' in a side ward. A mattress on the floor is the best way of preventing such patients from hurting themselves. At intervals check to see that all is well. Any remaining drugs or injection equipment have to be removed and locked safely away. Hours or a day later the patients will be off again to find more drugs in a never-ending circle of events. The only hope is for them to be persuaded to attend a drug-dependency unit.

When caring for the hardened addicts the nurse should be constantly aware of the possibility that they may be hepatitis B carriers. If they are, then any contact with their blood could be hazardous if she has a minute wound on her hand. Precautions are therefore essential (e.g. the wearing of plastic gloves), placing blood samples in additional sealed containers and disposing carefully of sharps.

DRUNKS

No accident and emergency department would be quite the same without drunks. They will always exist, so rules must apply when dealing with them:

1. Never simply 'label' a patient as a drunk. Each one must be thoroughly examined to rule out other conditions and injuries.
2. If a drunk has a head injury, he is just as likely to become

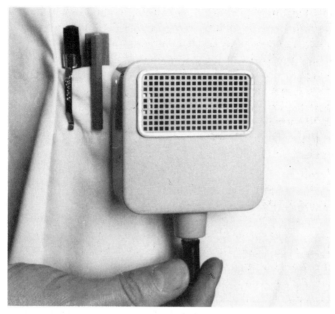

Fig. 157. *An alarm system in use at Whiston Hospital. If in any danger the nurse pulls the black peg and an alarm sounds in a central console to summon help.*

seriously ill as is a person who is sober and will, therefore, still require careful observation throughout the stay.

3. The aggressive drunk must be isolated from other patients receiving treatment, especially from children, who are easily frightened.

4. If available, a cubicle or sectioned-off area should be used where there is a minimum of furniture for the patient to damage, or to injure himself on.

5. If possible the patient should lie on a mattress on the floor for safety.

6. A nurse should be present all the time so that the patient cannot harm himself or others.

7. If you even *think* that violence may occur, get help at once to stand by in case of trouble. Do your utmost to be in a position where you have an escape route (nothing between you and the door) and have a friend within shouting distance. A simple alarm system is very helpful (Fig. 157).

8. If treatment is refused, in whole or part, or any untoward event occurs, such as violence or missing property, get it down in writing. If a colleague is there so much the better; in this way you will have something concrete on your side in case of litigation.

COMMON AND IMPORTANT POISONS WITH THEIR SPECIFIC TREATMENT

Aspirin. Aspirin is a dangerous drug, especially in small children. It is more likely to be lethal if the patient is experiencing tinnitus and treatment must not be delayed. Some people like to add sodium bicarbonate to the washout water, and sometimes to follow this by activated charcoal. A saline drip will be required after the washout. A specimen of blood can be taken to estimate the serum salicylates.

Iron. Iron is very dangerous to small children. This fact is not often realized by parents. Desferrioxamine is given, both down the stomach tube after washout (5 g) and intramuscularly (2 g). This is a chelating agent rendering the iron harmless.

Paracetamol. If large quantities of paracetamol have been absorbed cysteamine, N-acetylcysteine or methionine can be administered to help prevent liver damage.

Barbiturates. With barbiturate poisoning an intravenous infusion will be set up and a specimen of blood will be taken to estimate serum barbiturate levels. The patient's respirations will have to be observed carefully and intermittent positive-pressure ventilation instituted if necessary.

Benzodiazepines. The benzodiazepine group includes diazepam, chlordiazepoxide, nitrazepam and others. These drugs are very commonly taken, but do not have any particularly nasty side-effects. Care consists of clearing the airway until the patient 'wakes up'.

Turps substitute (white spirit), petrol and paraffin. With turps, petrol and paraffin the main danger is inhalation of the fumes, causing damage to the lungs. No stomach washout or ipecachuana is given. Instead, administer demulcents. A chest radiograph may be required and the patient will have to be observed closely for the distressed respirations of pulmonary oedema.

Disinfectants, bleach. Disinfectants and bleach form a rather diverse group which can vary from mildly irritant to highly corrosive. As a general rule no washout or emetic is given, the substance just being diluted with milky drinks.

Tricyclic antidepressants such as amitriptyline. The main danger with tricyclics is cardiac arrhythmia; monitoring will therefore be required even in seemingly fit patients.

Phenothiazines such as prochlorperazine or chlorpromazine. Extrapyramidal side-effects, such as spasm of face or eye muscles, can be particularly nasty for the patient when large doses of phenothiazines are taken. Relief, however, can be quickly achieved by administering a drug such as benztropine.

Morphine, pethidine, heroin, pentazocine, dextropropoxyphene. With all the drugs of the morphine group and others listed above, reversal can be achieved quickly with naloxone 0.4 mg, intravenously or intramuscularly. With dextropropoxyphene the initial dose of naloxone will be 1.2–2.4 mg. This can also be given as a test dose in an unconscious patient if poisoning by the above drugs is suspected.

Paraquat. Paraquat, a weedkiller, is not necessarily fatal unless the highly concentrated industrial form has been taken. A grey, sludgelike suspension of Fuller's earth and mannitol can be left in the stomach after a washout in an attempt to render it harmless.

Cyanide. Although strictly controlled, cyanide is still used in industry and accidents can happen. Kelocyanor by rapid intravenous injection immediately followed by 50% dextrose is the treatment of choice. If this fails, sodium nitrite and sodium thiosulphate can be tried. Speed of action is essential.

Magic mushrooms

In some parts of the UK including Merseyside where I live, a form of mushroom called magic mushroom (*Psilocybe semilanceata*) can be found growing. These are used by children and youths for 'kicks', but can also induce adverse effects and the youngsters finish up in hospital with hallucinations.

Treatment is by routine stomach emptying and symptomatic care. The effects should have disappeared by the next day, but the problem still remains of the patient's future course with drugs.

Parents and social workers working in harmony may be able to help.

Glue sniffing (solvent abuse)

This has become more a problem over the last few years. It mainly affects teenage youths. Typically, they put some glue such as Evo Stick into a plastic bag, place the bag round the nose and mouth, and breathe in the vapours. They quickly become 'high' on this, doing crazy things and may even become unconscious. The majority of cases never see an accident and emergency department, but there have been deaths, and the dangerous effects on health and relationships with other people are very sad indeed. A proportion of the youths will also take or have taken other types of drugs.

Care consists of looking after the airway until the acute effects of the solvent have worn off. The patient will sometimes have to be restrained if he is 'high'.

Social workers may sometimes be able to help with the problem in the long term as long as help is forthcoming from the youth's parents. However, it is a terrible problem with few clear answers.

FURTHER READING

Leech, K. (1983) *What everyone should know about drugs*. London: Sheldon Press.
Morton, A. (1983) Solvent abuse. *Nursing Mirror*: Supplement, 157:24(14 December).
Poisoning, *Nursing*, 1:15 (July) 668–671.
Westermeyer, J. (1976) *A primer on chemical dependency: a clinical guide to alcohol and drug problems*. Baltimore: Williams & Wilkins Co.

12   Soft tissue infections

The care of abscesses can be an intriguing subject and the relief afforded to the patient can be immense. The infected hand is especially challenging, requiring delicate, timely, yet purposeful attention, balanced with active exercises at the correct time. Poor treatment can result in 'wrecked machinery'.

GENERAL POINTS

Delay in attendance

A patient with an infection will often wait several days before seeking medical advice, hoping that it will ease and go away of its own accord. Many are extremely loath to attend until the pain finally drives them to us, often after one or even two sleepless nights. The scene can be likened to the dentist's surgery, many patients putting off regular attendances because of fear, until the unrelenting pain of toothache finally drives them eagerly to the dentist's door. The very fact that a patient has had a sleepless night with the pain almost always indicates that the abscess is ready for incision and this is a useful point to bear in mind.

Recognition

The standard features of any infection are as follows:

1. Pain, aching or throbbing in nature
2. Tenderness
3. Swelling
4. Local redness of the skin (erythema)
5. Increased local heat
6. Loss of function of the part concerned
7. Initially, the tissues feel hard and more firm than usual. Later, as pus develops, fluctuation will be found

Sometimes the infection will spread to the lymphatic vessels causing lymphangitis and to the local glands causing lymphadenitis. Spread through the subcutaneous tissues is called 'cellulitis'.

General effects such as raised temperature along with all its sequels can also occur. If the infection is in the hand or fingers, flexion may be noted at nearby joints; this is especially true of tendon sheath infections. It is the body's way of relaxing the tissues. Look at the way the patient walks in; if he has a hand infection, for instance, the hand is held up to the chest and there will be severe pain. If, on the other hand, the arm hangs down at the side, the pain cannot be too bad. Look at the patient's face; do you see pain and anxiety or a normal expression?

Organisms found

In swabs taken from soft tissue infections, you will find that the following organisms occur. If it is a hand infection, *Staphylococcus* is seen in the majority of instances, and *Streptococcus* occasionally. Now and then you may see *E. coli* and mixed infections. With infections round the anus, *E. coli* are found in about half the cases, the remainder being once again *Staphylococcus* and others. A high proportion of the staphylococci, somewhere in the region of 50 per cent, will be resistant to penicillin. With streptococci, penicillin will be effective.

History

While treating your patient it is very helpful to talk, not merely for social reasons, but to find out how and why the patient has acquired the infection. Ask if he remembers an injury or if he is a nail-biter (Fig. 158). Has the patient had any previous infections? Does he manicure? You will be surprised from time to time by the strange answers. In general, many patients are afraid to give the doctor information or do not hear the questions very well; in such instances the patient will be pleased to have the opportunity of speaking to you. It is also advisable to talk about his occupation, from the point of view of both diagnosis and prevention of food contamination. Ask if there is any history of previous infections anywhere in the body; if there is, bear in mind the possibility of diabetes and test accordingly.

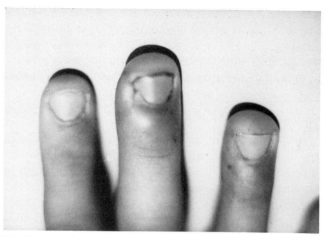

Fig. 158. *The typical nails of a nail-biter. Note the early paronychia in the middle finger.*

HAND INFECTIONS

Rest and elevation

With a hand infection, rest must be enforced. This can be done in several ways depending on the severity of the case. With lesser infections, for instance an early paronychia, no immobilization will be required. The patient is just advised not to allow the hand to remain dependent or do any heavy work until the pain eases. Alternatively, the patient's arm can be placed in a triangular sling to keep it elevated and out of use. On the ward a nurse can see every few minutes that the patient is doing the right thing. This is not so with accident and emergency work. When your patients get home, a substantial number will alter the treatment in some way. With hand injuries this tends to involve taking the hand out of any sling which has been applied and using it to do the odd task. Bearing this in mind, if the infection is severe and you do not want the patient to use it at all, there is a lot to be said for enclosing the whole hand in a 'boxing glove' type of dressing. A plaster back slab or splint is rarely necessary unless there is an infective tenosynovitis. When the patient is at home, the arm may be easier in the position mentioned in Chapter 9, for patients with Colles' fracture. This is with the arm resting on a cushion on the arm of a chair so that it is supported high in the air, thus easing throbbing and swelling.

Some patients with more severe infections, especially strepto-coccal ones, may require rest in bed, at home or as in-patients.

Release of pus and application of dressings

The time from onset of the symptoms to full maturation of the abscess varies tremendously with the individual conditions. Incision either too early or too late can have a profound effect on the patient, increasing the pain and spreading the infection further. As mentioned earlier, most will wait until they have at least one sleepless night because of the pain. You will find that the abscess is usually ready for incision after this 'bad' night.

The equipment required for incision of an abscess is as follows:

1. A standard sterile dressing pack
2. Sterile towels and clips
3. Lotions such as Savlon and Hibitane in spirit, for cleaning skin
4. Local anaesthetic, if used
5. Syringe and needles for the above
6. Ethyl chloride spray, if used
7. Small receiver
8. Bard Parker handle and blade
9. Toothed dissecting forceps
10. Sinus forceps
11. Scissors
12. Probe
13. Curette
14. Fine curved mosquito forceps
15. Spencer Wells artery forceps
16. Material for a pack, or a drain
17. Swab for the laboratory
18. Extra gauze and thick gamgee pads

Perhaps the nurse's major role is once again one of explaining what is about to happen, combined with reassurance. An abscess is a very painful thing and the patient will be very anxious not to suffer any more pain while it is being treated. The method of anaesthesia used will be an individual choice. A ring block is satisfactory for some distal infections, such as a paronychia, but a general anaesthetic is the ideal method for the majority of the more serious cases.

Many decry the use of ethyl chloride. I say it has an extremely valuable place in accident and emergency infections, as long as it is used for the correct type of case, and that it is used correctly. Many think that one squirt will last forever and the result is little better than torture for the patient. The correct method is first to explain its use to the patient and, especially with children, to show how it works, first on yourself and then on the patient's good limb. This will build up confidence. Let the part be cleaned and towelled and be sure that the doctor is ready to start. Next spray the site to be incised until the skin goes white; encouragement, of course, must be given to the patient throughout the procedure. The operator will then have about 15–30 seconds in which to complete the task before sensitivity returns. The method is ideal for the following:

1. A fairly small paronychia
2. An apical abscess
3. The removal of a nail with pus underneath
4. The removal of some splinters
5. Many of the miscellany of superficial lesions seen in the hand

A useful additive to ethyl chloride, or even for use on its own, is Entonox, although this will have to be commenced a good two minutes before the procedure starts.

Types of hand infection

Paronychia. The most common of all is paronychia which comprises about 80 per cent of all hand infections seen. Pus collects round the nail fold; it is often seen in patients who bite their nails (see Fig. 158). At incision, the subcutaneous blister of pus is deroofed and the base of the nail explored to ensure that all pus is released. When pus is under the nail, the proximal portion of the nail is cut away with scissors to allow adequate drainage. With an apical abscess, pus collects under the distal part of the pulp and nail. This is easily released by cutting a V out of the nail and

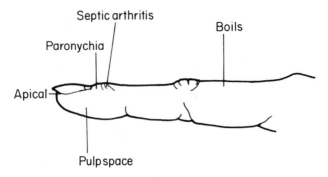

Fig. 159. *Common sites of infection in the fingers.*

deroofing the abscess underneath (see Fig. 160). Pulp space infections require skilful care if osteomyelitis of the terminal phalanx is to be avoided. This is because of the anatomy of the deep structures of the finger tip (Fig. 161). As you can see from the figure the artery passes through fibrous septa in the pulp space. If the infection causes increased pressure in one of these spaces, it is easy to see how the blood supply to the distal part of the terminal phalanx can be cut off and the infection spread to the bone. Timely and adequate incision must be made as soon as pus develops.

Boils and carbuncles. These will be seen on the hairy part of the back of the hand and will discharge of their own accord. Sometimes the pus will require 'helping out' and the lesion will heal more quickly if the loose slough is removed with forceps.

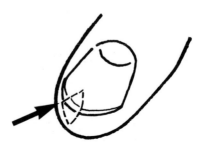

Fig. 160. *The area to cut away to deroof an apical abscess.*

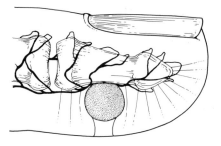

Fig. 161. *How pus in the pulp space can damage the blood vessels supplying the bone.*

Infection of the web spaces. The web spaces between the digits can become infected following trauma and the swelling is seen to push the two adjacent digits apart. Deroofing of any blister and/or small incision on the palmar side may be necessary.

Palmar infections. Like web infections, palmar infections are caused mainly by trauma, commonly a penetrating wound or splinter. Incision is made over the subcuticular part of the abscess to deroof it or over the site of maximum tenderness. With both palmar and pulp space infections in particular, 'collar studding' is very likely to be present (Fig. 162). This is where there is a deep cavity with a small connection to an obvious superficial collection of pus. Release of the superficial collection only is of no use at all. The connection between the two must be sought and enlarged.

With the opening of all abscesses, the incision should be of adequate size. Minute 'nicks' are generally of little use because

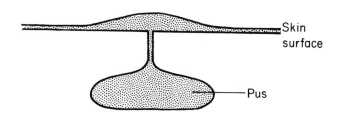

Fig. 162. *A 'collar-stud' abscess. Never be fooled.*

they will close up within a few hours. If there is any danger of closure, either the wound can be cut at the edges, so that it gapes or a small pack can be inserted. Beware of the 'cork in the bottle' effect of packing tightly. It looks great at the time of incision with blood and pus still seeping through, but after about an hour everything clogs up, retaining all the pus. Things can be made a lot worse by the use of glycerine magnesium sulphate paste which sets like cement (Fig. 163). Sometimes an antibiotic cream (fusidic acid) is inserted into the cavity after evacuation of the pus and left for several days. Otherwise a dry dressing is all that should be necessary. A comparatively new substance, Debrisan, which consists of minute dry porous beads which absorb exudate, may hold promise for the future, but I have not had enough experience of its use at this stage. The frequency of dressing will vary with the patient, although almost all patients should return the following day for a dressing to ensure that all is well. An important question which you should ask the patient is 'Is there any improvement?' Even if it still hurts (which it probably will), so long as it is getting better all is well. Following incision the patient should have little or no throbbing pain and should also have had a reasonable night's sleep. If the hand is still throbbing and the patient is not sleeping another incision may be necessary, so ask the doctor to see the patient. The first day after incision is the time to start encouraging

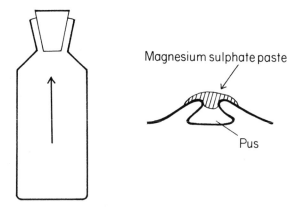

Fig. 163. *The 'cork in the bottle' effect of a wick soaked in magnesium sulphate paste.*

the patient to do active exercises with the fingers. Little movement will show at this stage but the patient has plenty of time at home to practice and as the days go by things should return to normal. As the dressings are done, any hard, thick skin should be cut or peeled away. The removal of this skin will aid rehabilitation and also help drainage if no formal incision has been done. When the dressings are done, a full aseptic technique must be strictly adhered to, so that further contamination is not made. However, when applying the final dressing, use fingers so that the dressing can be accurately positioned. Never simply wrap the dressing round; it is far better to zig-zag it over the site of the incision so that there will be maximum absorbent material where it is required (Fig. 164). In the acute stages try not to use tube-gauze. All too frequently this is applied far too tightly causing constriction and therefore more pain for the patient (Fig. 165). A bandage enclosing two fingers is far more comfortable. Also, avoid the mistake of applying too bulky a dressing, thus limiting the exercises which the patient can perform.

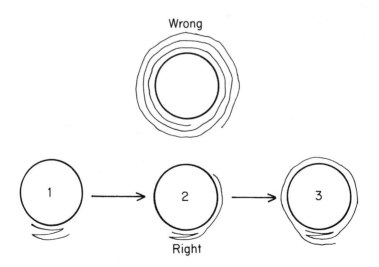

Fig. 164. *Instead of simply wrapping a dressing round a finger it is best to zig-zag it over the wound first. This will give the maximum of absorbent material where it is required.*

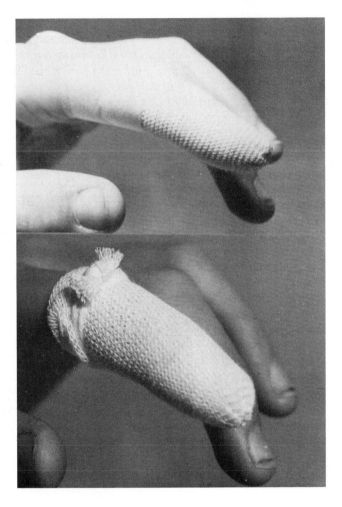

Fig. 165. *If tube-gauze is applied, stick it to the finger. This will cause far less constriction and pain than tying it.*

AXILLARY ABSCESSES

Although at first sight you may think that a sling is of use here, the patient usually wishes the arm to be away from the side of the chest to ease the pain. Rest is therefore confined to stopping work and using the arm as little as possible. At home the patient will find some relief if the elbow is at rest on the arm of a chair.

Before any incision is attempted the axillary hair should be shaved and the whole area washed as it will be smelly and sweaty. The patient should be positioned lying flat with his hand on top of the head; this will give the operator a good view of the axilla. In carefully selected cases ethyl chloride, possibly plus Entonox or pethidine, is completely satisfactory for incision, giving the experienced operator ample time to make an incision, open the abscess up thoroughly and express the pus with sinus forceps. Advanced cases may require a general anaesthetic. Surgifix or one of the conforming tapes are the ideal methods of keeping the dressing in position (Fig. 166). Rehabilitation is no problem; the patient will soon start to move the limb again once the pain subsides.

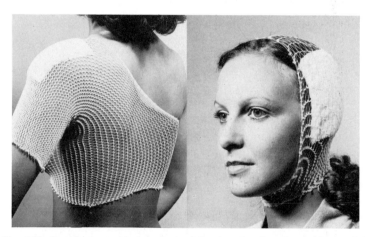

Fig. 166. *Surgifix is an ideal method of keeping dressings in position and is especially useful for awkward places.*

PERIANAL ABSCESSES

In a substantial number of cases the perianal abscess has pointed and/or started to discharge by the time the patient arrives in the unit. You can hardly blame the patient for putting things off as long as possible; I am sure that most readers of this book would not like to attend with an abscess in such an awkward place! While attending to your patient he should be lying prone with a pillow under the chest and the head resting on his arms. Wash and shave the region near the abscess. In most instances the doctor will want to carry out a rectal examination. Unless the abscess is already pointing, it will usually be necessary for the incision to be made under general anaesthesia. Once asleep, the patient will have to be turned onto one side or placed in the lithotomy position. Dressings will be held in place once again with Netalast. Several hours may pass before the patient will feel well enough to go home.

I have found the best form of aftercare for these patients is to see them again on the day following incision. If all is well when the dressing is done, give them a supply of gauze and gamgee to take home. Ask the patient to have a warm bath with an antiseptic or salt in it, two or three times a day. Afterwards dab the part dry and apply a dry dressing and pad. The patient will then only require review again in about a week to ensure that all has healed well. I have never known a patient not to do well on this regimen.

INFECTED SEBACEOUS CYSTS

Many people have cysts all their lives and have no trouble from them. Occasionally they can become infected. Some, if treated early, respond well to antibiotics and settle down again to their usual quiet state. Others will require simple incision and drainage to settle down. Note that no attempt is made to remove the cyst at this stage. These cysts are commonly seen round the face, head and neck, so that once again Surgifix is the ideal method of holding a dressing in position. If the patient does not want to wear this, use tape such as Blenderm to make the dressing as socially acceptable as possible. If the cyst is behind the ear, strapping can sometimes be applied carefully so that the dressing is hardly seen.

INFECTED INGROWING TOENAILS

Infected ingrowing toenail is a chronic condition which should not be treated on an accident and emergency unit. It can, however, have an acute stage when it becomes infected and the patient turns up for help.

Antibiotics will be needed to help clear the infection up and the patient must be referred back to a general practitioner for long-term treatment.

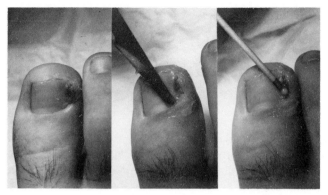

Fig. 167. *After cleaning, petroleum jelly is applied round the area of granulation. A moistened silver nitrate stick is then applied to the granulated area. The petroleum jelly prevents it damaging normal tissue.*

Local care

First, clean up the mess which usually presents because in many instances the patient will have had no form of dressing over the toe, the pus just being allowed to discharge into the sock. An excess of granulation tissue is often seen at one corner of the nail. Remove any crusting from this with care so that it does not bleed. Cut out a small wedge of nail from near the granulation tissue; this does nothing to help the nail in the long term, but while there is an infection present it will aid drainage and ease pressure on the tender swollen tissue. Smear petroleum jelly round the granulation tissue and apply a moistened silver nitrate stick to the granulation (Fig. 167); it will immediately turn a greyish colour. Cover the whole with a dry dressing and use tube-gauze bandage. Instruct the patient that, when at home, he should raise the foot on pillows and not wear slippers or a sock, otherwise pressure will continue. The patient is then referred back to a general practitioner for daily dressings until the condition settles down again.

13 Dealing with the aggressive, difficult or psychiatric patient

In this chapter I would like to tell you how to deal with aggression, which can vary from complaints and abusive language, through threatening behaviour to outright physical violence. In many instances it is important to realize that dealing with the first two situations sensibly will reduce the number of times that physical violence is reverted to. To understand the subject a little more, let us list the main causes of aggressive and violent behaviour on an accident and emergency department:

- Alcohol
- Drugs
- Psychiatric conditions
- Long waiting times
- Rowdy behaviour of a group of youths not handled correctly
- Lack of communication
- Staff aggravating patients

From this list we can now formulate some general rules to help us prevent physical violence and cut down aggressive behaviour.

Alcohol is perhaps the major cause of our problems. A very high percentage of all patients who come into the accident and emergency department after 10 p.m. have taken it. I am not saying that they are drunk, but their thought processes are altered and they react differently to circumstances than a person who has had no drink at all. As an example of this, I can think of occasions when people I know have come into the department at night with injured relatives and have acted completely out of character because of alcohol; they have been very awkward in manner, complaining and rowdy. In fact in these circumstances it is easy to understand how if a young female nurse had been present who was not adept at handling drunks the situation could have become very unpleasant or even violent.

Some nurses, through no fault of their own, have an unfortunate knack of meeting awkward patients 'head on' as if to do battle. This leaves the patient with no opportunity to side track and calm down without losing face. Whether we like the idea or not, in almost every incident of violence in the accident and emergency department, the patient had *not* come to us with the idea of beating up nurses. They or their friends either want some sort of help or have been brought to the department against their will and simply want to get out. We can usually avoid physical violence by the way we handle them. For instance, at first it is often far better to humour a drunk, reverting to firm behaviour if tact does not work. A smile, a steady hand and perhaps a few words like 'Oh come on John, let's get you safely home, you'll feel better in the morning' is often a far better approach than standing firm with a face and voice like thunder, trying to push a drunk around and making him look foolish (Fig. 168).

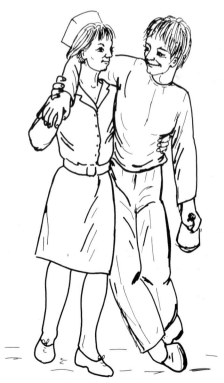

Fig. 168. *The happy drunk.*

An added precaution is to ask for help to be brought into the department if there is a situation in which you think there may be trouble. Do not wait for the situation to get out of hand before calling. I feel that this point is not fully grasped by many night-time managers. The presence of a male member of staff just seen nearby can often act as a deterrent to verbal and physical violence.

Drugs and alcohol often go hand in hand especially during an evening, enhancing each others effect and making the patient one of the most complex problems for the accident and emergency nurse. However, despite all the difficulties, such patients usually submit to our treatment fairly quietly with tactful handling by ourselves, friends or relatives.

Groups of youths often wander into the department when one of their number has some fairly trivial injury. Their shabby unkempt appearance and boisterous manner tend to be very out of place in the hospital environment. When handling them go easy to start off with, use words like 'come on now lads, this is a hospital waiting room, I've got sick people over there and this noise will upset them'. Something like this will usually work: a friendly but firm reminder that they are overdoing things will not instantly get their 'backs up'. Many fool about in the streets like that all the time so they do not realize that they are being particularly antisocial. If the disturbance continues, isolate the leader; they are obviously out for trouble and need firm handling. Depending on your own assessment of the situation either get the hospital security men or the police in to move them straight away. Ordinary members of the public and especially children or sick people should not be subjected to such disturbances. Only try moving a group like that if you are sure that you can cope with violence on your own if things go wrong. Remember also that if a group of youths have been cleared from the accident and emergency department for causing a disturbance, they quite frequently go snooping round the hospital instead of simply going home. Staff cars, windows, wards and storerooms can all take a toll of their wrath. It is better if they are escorted off the premises completely.

Having to wait a long time is a cause of much frustration for patients and relatives, especially if the patients are in pain. Quite often those in the waiting room do not see the serious accidents coming in and therefore, have no way of knowing that staff are busy. So, bear in mind that an occasional shout of explanation into the waiting room may save much aggression coming your way. (It may even clear the waiting room!)

Some particularly difficult patients or relatives try to get seen quickly by using the waiting room as a stage. They pick on a nurse or clerk and try to queue-jump by bluffing their way through with aggressive language and stirring up the audience. Such people should not be allowed to get away with it.

The best approach is for a senior member of the staff to go out, sit next to them and quietly explain why they are waiting; never give in just for a quiet life.

Let us next consider some general points:

- On night duty, especially on a small department, stock up in advance so that your colleagues do not have to go to a quiet dark or isolated area. Attack is far less likely in busy well-lit areas.
- Call for help to stand by on the department to prevent trouble starting and to be there in good time if it does occur; do not wait for the fists to fly.
- Never be on your own with a patient if you are unsure of him.
- If trouble 'rumbles' you will be less vulnerable as one of a group; a nurse on her own is far more likely to be attacked.
- Keep between the patient and the door when tending a patient in a room, you then have an escape route and can easily call for help.
- Wear an alarm if available (see Fig. 157).

Deterring an attacker

Let us now presume that all of the foregoing advice has failed and things have gone too far, an attack is occurring or the patient is closing in on you.

As a rule nurses are not aggressive people and this could be their downfall. It is difficult for them to suddenly alter from being caring people to people who are going to hurt another. But this is what must happen; it must be thought of beforehand and planned, otherwise you will be useless when the situation arises.

If you are female, then you will probably be weaker than the patient who attacks you, purely because of the way you are built. You cannot and must not try to match the strength of your attacker, the odds would be against you. Instead you must rely on your skill and cunning to surprise your attacker, hurt him and make a quick escape to help.

Your main stumbling block could be in your own mind, still thinking of your attacker as a patient. However, as soon as he has shown physical violence towards you, the nurse–patient relationship must be forgotten. What is to come may seem like a catalogue of 'dirty tricks' but what you are facing is physical violence, a stage of no return, where you either hurt the attacker or get hurt yourself.

Methods of possible attack are obviously far too numerous for me to go into in any detail. All I can do in the limited space is to mention broad principles which can be built on by reading or night school classes if you are interested. The local police may be interested in giving a group of you some coaching, and if all else fails practising a few moves with a friend is better than nothing.

Firstly, you have to call for help; noise will sometimes tend to scare an assailant away. Next you have to surprise him with sudden, severe pain so that his grip on you will be released. To do this you just have to remember the more delicate parts of a person's body (Fig. 169) and hit him hard with whatever part of you he has not got hold of. Remember, now is not the time for nursing, now is the time to hurt. Be ruthless in an attempt to save yourself from possibly severe injury.

Frontal attack. If this occurs try to aim for the sensitive areas under the nose or the eyeballs. Hit him with either your fingers or items you may carry such as pens and keys. Failing that, bring your knee up *hard* into his groin. That should bring even the largest assailant to his knees long enough for you to escape and run. Remember, I am not telling you how to fight, simply how to make a get-away to help which should be very fast in coming.

Attack from the rear. This situation is more difficult and frightening because you have been surprised. However, once again your only hope (unless you are an expert in unarmed combat) is to hurt your attacker so that the grip will be released and you can run. Aim for the sensitive parts of the body, and in this instance the front of the shins could be accessible. Dig the back of your heel into him and scrape it right down the front (Fig. 170).

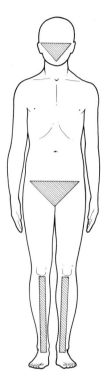

Fig. 169. *Where to hurt an attacker.*

Restraining a patient on a trolley

Another awkward situation is where you have a patient on a trolley who becomes violent (Fig. 171) and because of his condition has to be restrained. While waiting for the police, consider the following hints:

• Being near to the feet is a danger, especially if the patient still has shoes on. Always try to take a restless patient's shoes off as soon as possible to avoid injury to staff.
• Remember that the patient's head can also be a weapon, so do not bend over him too closely, you could be butted, bitten or spat on.

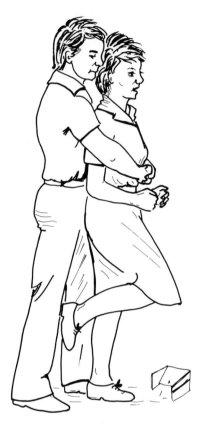

Fig. 170. *With an attack from the rear, try to dig your heel into the shin and push down.*

- The most common injury is caused by a patient who more or less waves his arms about struggling and hits a nurse in the face. It is rare for a confused patient to deliberately aim a punch at a nurse.

To avoid all the above, adequate numbers of staff are required. One person will be required to hold one of the patient's arms by the wrist. It can be held down at the patient's side or up by his head. Holding both the wrist and a cot side together saves energy and can be done by even a small nurse (Fig. 172). The legs are more of a problem; sometimes they can be left alone to thrash

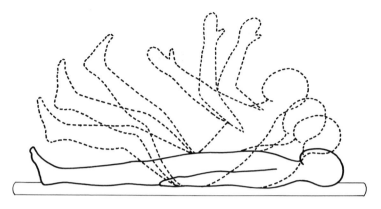

Fig. 171. *Danger areas with a restless patient on a trolley.*

about as long as everyone is out of the way. At other times at least two more people will be required to press down on the knees.

Münchausens

Not everyone who enters our department with a complaint will be genuine. Some have the express desire to try to fool you into giving them drugs or obtaining their admission into hospital. I list

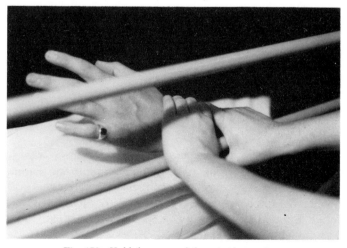

Fig. 172. *Hold the arm and the cot side together.*

below some of the pointers which should 'ring alarm bells' in your mind.

Injection marks on the patient's body
Numerous scars on the patient's abdomen from operations
Renal colic
Chest pains
Haematuria if you do not see the patient actually pass it
No next of kin or relatives who cannot be contacted
An unusual story
Exaggeration of symptoms (you will know this by experience)
No fixed abode
A job which takes the patient all over the country
A patient who becomes agitated or aggressive if his details are questioned

Many will go from one hospital to the other around the country gaining either admission or drugs, it being almost a way of life to them. It is important that if you come across these patients that details are telephoned to other hospitals in the area so that they do not hoodwink them. Often these patients will recover suddenly, get dressed and walk out if they feel that you are onto them. Until you are sure of your facts do not confront these patients with what you suspect. The local police are a great help because they are able to check up in a few minutes whether a particular person lives at a given address. Pain-killing drugs should be withheld from such patients in spite of their protestations, while quick enquiries are made. If their story checks we have to give it. In order to cut down the number of times such patients trick junior staff it is useful to have a list of their various aliases and a description of them and their complaints.

REFUSAL OF TREATMENT

In a ward setting, you care every day for patients who want to be treated and who signify this fact by their very presence. This is not always true of the accident and emergency department. Hardly a day goes by without someone refusing some or all of the treatment offered. Below I have broadly categorized the patients, because the approach varies considerably.

Adults

Adults have a perfect right to refuse any treatment. Although it is best in such instances to ask them to sign a form to this effect, it is by no means compulsory. In all cases, however, you should ensure that the reasons for the treatment have been adequately explained to them. Often coaxing and a sympathetic explanation by a colleague will do the trick.

Psychiatric patients

Psychiatric patients like any others have likes, dislikes and opinions, and these should be honoured as with any mentally fit patient. However, if the patient's decision involves danger to self or others and discussion has proved fruitless, the patient will have to be detained.

Problems occasionally arise with mentally disturbed patients when they wish to leave the department before they have been seen by a doctor, or while waiting for a psychiatrist to arrive.

Although at first this might appear to be a complicated legal situation, in practical reality it is quite straight-forward. If you think that a patient is a danger to self or others then do your best to detain him until a doctor says that he is safe to go. If you do not have the physical capability to detain him, then call the police to help you. To allow such a patient to simply walk away is negligent.

Precise legal details will be found in the Mental Health Act 1983, under section 5 *Application in respect of patient already in hospital*, (4) *Nurses' holding power.*

This situation, however, is rare; tact and persuasion usually win through.

Children

With children the problem is straight-forward. If the parents are present or give consent over the phone, the treatment can be carried out. If they cannot be contacted, important items, such as suturing which cannot wait, should be carried out, but nothing like anti-tetanus toxoid, penicillin or a general anaesthetic can be given until the parents are contacted.

In an emergency in which the parents or guardian cannot be contacted, the physician or surgeon will take the responsibility for treatment. If necessary, the child will be made a ward of court in the UK.

A situation commonly occurs in which the child does not want to have an injection. If all coaxing and reasoning with the child are fruitless, avoid the situation becoming prolonged for more than a minute or two. Get the assistance of one or possibly two other nurses to restrain the child tactfully while the most experienced quickly gives the injection. Never lie by saying 'It won't hurt' and always try to make 'pals' again with the child afterwards. Most children will have been surprised that it hurt so little, and if befriended will make a far better response if the situation occurs in the future.

Drunks

A drunken patient who refuses treatment creates an awkward situation. My own opinion on this matter is that if a drunk says 'no', a reasonable explanation should be tried first, especially if the treatment is fairly important. Have a witness present while you do this. If the patient still says 'no', ask for a signature on a refusal form. Whether or not the patient signs it, let him go. The alternative to this is violence towards the nursing staff, which should be prevented.

THE DISTURBED PSYCHIATRIC PATIENT

The disturbed psychiatric patient can take up more nurses' time than the most serious road traffic accident. This fact is realized by most who work in the accident and emergency department, but by few outsiders. A disturbed psychiatric patient can also upset children and other physically ill patients far more than any visually unpleasant casualty. This fact is realized by few outsiders and seldom acted on. Your approach to the patient varies with each individual problem. However, while waiting for psychiatric help, the following guide lines can be given:

1. Try to have the patient isolated, away from the noise and activity of the general patients.

2. Remove any equipment which may be in the area so that the patient cannot damage it or use it to hurt himself.
3. Make an immediate decision as to whether any accompanying relatives have an inflammatory or sedating effect on the patient. If the effect is good let them stay.
4. If possible, let one senior nurse build up some form of relationship with the patient.
5. If appropriate, get close to the patient and listen to what he has to say, making just the occasional comment.
6. If, despite tactful coaxing, violence looks likely, summon adequate numbers of suitable staff so that neither patient nor staff are likely to be injured. Arrangements made at a local level probably already exist for such events.
7. The police must be summoned in cases of severe psychiatric violence in the accident and emergency department. This situation is thankfully an extreme rarity. Most instances involving the police start outside in the community, the police travelling to hospital in the ambulance with the patient.
8. Drugs are not the only way of 'quietening' a patient, but if necessary should be given quickly and in adequate doses.

EXAGGERATION OF SYMPTOMS AND HYSTERIA

All patients will respond differently to a painful stimulus by showing varying amounts of pain or discomfort. But, as an extra complication, some patients will want to prolong, exaggerate or invent symptoms. The reasons for doing this include the following:

1. The chance of more compensation
2. Getting time off work
3. Seeking sympathy or attention
4. Loneliness

The big problem is how to decide where malingering ends and hysteria begins; it can be very difficult. A mixture of intuition and experience of the normal reaction and progress of a given injury are a nurse's only aids even if old notes are to hand.

Dangers also lie in wait for those who make this diagnosis too freely. Over the years I can think of several instances where patients have been proved right. This has almost always been with an unusual presentation of a disease or injury or where tests show nothing amiss. One example is the patient with chest pain who is sent home because nothing shows on an ECG and is brought in dead the next day! The only way to avoid missing something is to rule out other possibilities carefully first, even if the patient is 'well known' to the hospital.

True hysteria can manifest itself in a multitude of ways. A few of the more common presentations are overbreathing causing carpopedal spasm; pins and needles in the feet and hands; fits of a 'bizarre' nature, quite unlike any textbook descriptions; paralysis of an arm or leg and/or sensory disturbances which do not correctly fit into any anatomical boundaries. Various states of impaired consciousness can also occur, as can depressive and other psychiatric conditions.

FURTHER READING

Pisarick, G. (1981) Facing the violent patient, *Nursing*, 11:9 (September), 61–65.
Wright, B. (1983) Who are the regulars? *Nursing Times* 79:7.
Yoder, L. & Jones, S.L. (1982) The emergency room nurse and the psychiatric patient. *Journal of Psychosocial Nursing*, 20 (6 June), 22–28.

14 Eye and ENT injuries

THE EYE

FOREIGN BODIES

Many patients have a great fear of anything being done to their eyes and will be very apprehensive about what treatment awaits them. Efficient care depends on the patient's cooperation, which will only be forthcoming after an adequate explanation of what is to happen and reassurance that he will suffer little or no pain.

Positioning of the patient is very important; lying down with the head resting comfortably on a pillow is ideal. The operator must be able to stand at the patient's head and still have adequate lighting. Your very approach will also convey your ability to the patient, fumbling and indecisive fingers giving him little confidence in you. Before the eye is examined all patients should be asked how the injury occurred. In particular note any history which would entail the foreign body travelling at high speed, such as one incurred while using a grinding wheel, hammering metal or riding a motor bike. This should always draw your mind to the possibility of an intraocular foreign body. The entry wound can easily be overlooked and the patient may be almost symptomless at first. A radiograph will be essential for any patient with such a history.

All parts of the eye should be examined for foreign bodies, not merely the part in which the patient feels pain. During the examination foreign bodies in the eye may be invisible unless looked at from a particular angle. This is especially true if they lie over the pupil or a dark iris.

Everting the lower eyelid is easily done, but to evert the upper lid takes a little practice. Sometimes a small stick is necessary but in most instances the lid can be everted just using your fingers (Fig. 173). Stand behind the patient and hold onto the upper eyelashes with the thumb and index finger of the left hand. Ask the patient to look downwards. Press the tip of your right index finger onto the upper lid and push down; at the same time pull backwards with the left hand. When this is done the lid should evert easily and stay like that with only one hand holding it. Practise the technique on some of your friends until you are proficient.

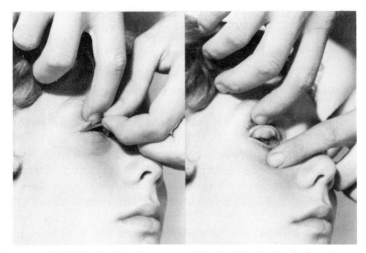

Fig. 173. *Everting the upper eyelid to look for foreign bodies.*

If nothing can be seen in the eye it should then be stained with a drop of fluorescein and the excess washed away. This will show up any scratching of the cornea and often a foreign body such as a fine white hair which was invisible beforehand.

Removal of the foreign body should always be attempted first with a moistened cotton wool 'bud'. If it rests on the cornea, local anaesthetic drops will be required. Amethocaine 1% is used and you will have to wait about 15 seconds for it to work. Warn your patient that, after insertion, the eye will sting for a few moments. If the foreign body will not move with the cotton bud, a sharp-pointed needle may have to be tried. This is a very delicate procedure which a nurse should not attempt until she is completely familiar with the technique required and has done it previously under adequate supervision.

After removal of the foreign body the doctor may require an antibiotic ointment and/or mydriatics to be placed in the eye. If local anaesthetic has been used the eye will require a pad, at least until the sensations have fully returned (a few hours).

Warn patients about the dangers of driving or operating machinery with only one eye in use. If removal has been difficult and amethocaine was necessary, mention that once the amethocaine has worn off the eye will once again become painful but that this is normal and should gradually ease. Many patients will gladly tolerate such discomfort as long as they know that it is 'normal'.

CORNEAL ABRASIONS

Abrasions are very commonly caused by foreign bodies and their removal, fingers being poked into the eye or a whole host of other comparatively trivial accidents such as catching the eye with a newspaper. The result of all these is damage to the cornea of varying severity.

These abrasions can often be seen if the eye is studied closely under a bright light. However, if a drop of fluorescein is placed in the eye, it will stain the abrasion bright yellow/green, showing it up clearly.

The majority of superficial abrasions will heal well with no after-effects. Care demands an antibiotic ointment, perhaps mydriatic drops and padding of the eye for a few days until the symptoms have eased. If any of your patients have a painful eye condition, advise them to go home, not back to work, where they will be a danger. Warn them against watching TV or using the 'good' eye too much, because movements of the good eye will be duplicated in the painful one, aggravating the pain. Advise them to lie down in a room with soft lighting, listening to records or the radio.

CHEMICAL BURNS

When any irritant or corrosive chemical is splashed into the eye, as often occurs in industry or schools, the first aid care is to wash the eye with running water. In my experience, by the time the patient reaches hospital this has been done in almost every instance. We must now continue the care by repeatedly washing out the affected eye with saline until relief is obtained. With children or very nervous adults amethocaine will be required beforehand so that you can gain access. When large amounts of fluid are required quickly, an intravenous infusion apparatus can be set up. This will run a good stream of sterile saline into the eye, and can be directed easily and is convenient to handle. Buffer solutions are also available if required for corrosive burns. After this, the eye will require staining so that the extent of the damage can be seen.

Nothing should delay the initial washout: no sitting in waiting rooms or filling in cards. Get on with it and ask questions later!

CONTACT LENSES

Occasionally a contact lens can become 'lost' and slip out of sight somewhere in the conjuctival sac. As lenses can only be worn for a certain number of hours each day, removal will become important. If they are left in, severe irritation will result. The patients sometimes have small suction devices which will aid removal. If not, the suction will have to be released by manipulation in order to remove the lens. Ask a friend who wears such lenses to show you how it is done.

Be alert to the possibility of the presence of lenses in unconscious patients.

WELDERS' 'FLASH'

Your patient will have been doing some welding during the past few hours without wearing his usual protective goggles or shield. Very severe irritation will be present in both eyes and they will be reddened. The patients have usually had the condition before and will walk in telling you the diagnosis. In most instances the condition will be cared for by instillation of anaesthetic drops and/or antibiotic ointment, plus covering the eyes with pads. By the next day the eyes will be greatly improved.

BLOW-OUT FRACTURE OF THE ORBIT

With a severe blow to the orbit, the pressure inside can be raised to such an extent that the thin bony floor or wall will fracture. As this occurs tissue such as an ocular muscle can be driven through the fracture into the sinus, becoming trapped (Fig. 174). Among other things the patient may complain of double vision; surgical emphysema can occur around the orbit if the patient blows the nose. If the patient is asked to look upwards the affected eye will not have as full a range of movement. A more common injury, also caused by a frontal blow to the eye, is hyphema (Fig. 175). This is a collection of blood in the anterior chamber. The patient will require rest and admission.

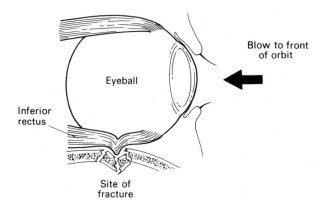

Fig. 174. *Blow-out fracture of the floor of the orbit.*

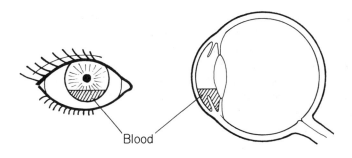

Fig. 175. *Hyphema: bleeding into the anterior chamber of the eye.*

RUST RING

Occasionally, after removal of a metallic corneal foreign body, a small ring is left in the cornea. If this occurs, the patient should be given antibiotic drops and sent to the ophthalmic surgeon who will be able to remove it far more easily in a couple of days time. This fact should be explained to the patient so that he does not mistakenly consider the doctor to be negligent.

EAR, NOSE AND THROAT

EPISTAXIS

A nose bleed is a very common problem. The patient, of no matter what age group, is often alarmed, thinking he is losing a dangerous amount of blood. Although serious blood loss can occur, this is the exception rather than the rule; the average loss only fills an eggcup. Predisposing causes of the condition include the patient picking or blowing the nose after a cold and hypertension.

The first essential in care, apart from resuscitation if the patient is shocked, is to reassure the patient that all will soon be well. If you are calm and authoritative, your very approach will give the patient confidence. Try the simple first-aid treatment first; it is surprising how few people know of it. Your patient should sit up on a trolley and lean forward. The head is tilted forwards and after clearing out any mounds of clot from the nostrils and pharynx the nose is pinched (Fig. 176) for about 10 minutes. Ask the patient to breathe through the mouth and not to talk or swallow anything. Loosen any tight clothing round the neck. The pulse and blood pressure should always be taken and occasionally the doctor will want to do blood investigations.

If the simple method advised above does not work the nose will have to be packed. Ask the patient not to cough or sneeze and explain that the pack will feel a little unpleasant. The patient's head should be resting comfortably on a pillow. Remove excesses of blood clot from the nose. Several forms of pack may be used. The commonest is plain petroleum jelly gauze or Calgitex. The exact technique is best shown at the bedside, but generally speaking the pack should be inserted in a zig-zag pattern (Fig. 177), using nasal dressing forceps under adequate vision. Afterwards have a look at the back of the throat to ensure that the blood is not simply trickling down the pharynx. If bleeding persists the ENT surgeon may wish to attempt re-packing using a balloon, to cauterize, to use a posterior nasal pack or, if all else fails, to take the patient to theatre to tie off one of the arteries supplying the nose.

FOREIGN BODIES IN THE NOSE AND EARS

Foreign bodies in the nose are seen almost exlusively in children and are limitless in their variety. Their presence is often not even

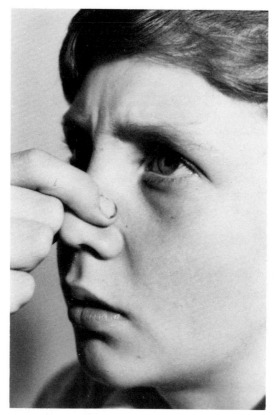

Fig. 176. *Pinching the nose to stop bleeding. To be effective pressure should continue for about ten minutes.*

suspected until a foul discharge starts.

One of the main nursing points to consider is that the casualty officer may well have only one chance to get the foreign body out with comparative ease: that is when the child first arrives and is happy. Repeated attempts with the child held insecurely will result in a frightened, crying, struggling child, making removal of the foreign body very difficult. In an accident and emergency department, where all the surroundings are strange and frightening to a child, taking the child away from its mother will mostly result in crying. Because of this it is best to leave the child on the mother's knee so that he will be comforted and feel safe. Instruct the mother

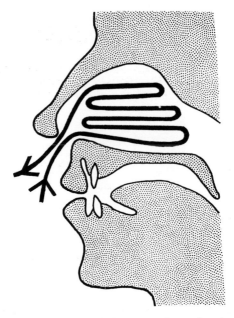

Fig. 177. *A method of insertion of a nasal pack.*

how to stop protesting arms and legs getting in the doctor's way and if necessary hold the child's head firmly yourself. Alternatively, if the parents are of no help, the child can be engulfed in a blanket and laid down or held by a nurse.

With foreign bodies in the ears, adults start to enter the picture. Pieces of cotton wool or the like may become 'lost' while the ears are being cleaned. If the patient is a child, the head will require firm support as mentioned above.

No matter where the foreign body is, remember the principle that 'attack' from the front of the object will tend to drive it further in. Ideally something should be passed around it so that it can be pulled out (Fig. 178).

FISH BONE IN THE THROAT

A bone lodged in the throat is a very uncomfortable condition causing the patient much distress. The bone is often difficult to see especially with a nervous and uncooperative patient. Radiographs may be required if the bone cannot be seen. In many instances the bone has merely scratched the mucosa 'on the way down' but the

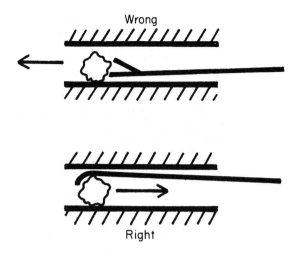

Fig. 178. *A foreign body can easily be driven further inwards by faulty technique.*

continuing severe discomfort makes the patient feel as though it
had lodged.

BLEEDING TOOTH SOCKET

If bleeding from a tooth socket has been severe and prolonged,
bear in mind the possibility of shock being present. It is not
unknown for a patient to have to be given an intravenous infusion
after a bad bleed.

First clean all the clot from the mouth and if necessary give a
brief mouthwash. Lay the patient down with the head resting on a
pillow. There must be a good light. Remove the clot from the
socket itself so that the bleeding point can be identified. Pack the
socket firmly with Calgitex, Sterispon or gauze soaked in adrenaline. Ask the patient to bite on this and leave him undisturbed,
lying down, for about half an hour. If unsuccessful then repeat;
only after a couple of attempts will suture of the socket become
necessary.

FURTHER READING

Seewoodhary, M. (1983) Common presentations in accident and emergency.
Nursing, 2:17 (September) 498–501.

15   Paediatric problems

In this short chapter I would like to draw together some of the major problems associated with children in an accident and emergency department. However, many more details of specific conditions will be found scattered through the book in specialist chapters.

Ideally, all injured children should be cared for by RSCNs in specialist children's hospitals. The ideal is, however, a 'pipe dream' and we must in the meantime do the best we can by improving what we already have by way of facilities, equipment and knowledge (Fig. 179).

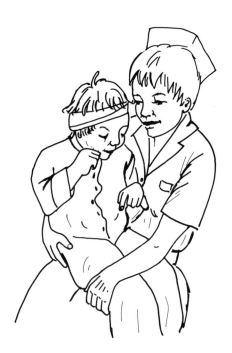

Fig. 179. *Even if you have poor facilities, kindness will stick in a child's mind.*

INFANTILE CONVULSIONS

In infantile convulsions, there are two problems, the child and the frantically upset parents. Quite understandably even in what is to us quite a minor case, the parents think that their baby may die. If the child is still 'fitting', attend at once to the airway. Also, remember that with very young the fitting can seem to be more of a tremor than a true fit.

Undress the child and take the rectal or axillary temperature. In the majority of cases this will be raised, possibly due to an upper respiratory tract infection or sometimes something more sinister. If it is raised, leave the child uncovered and cool with a fan or by tepid sponging. Many parents want to keep wrapping the child up 'so that he doesn't catch cold', so explain your actions.

Rectal diazepam (Valium) is frequently given if the fit continues and in most cases is very effective.

Initially, while the child is 'fitting', it may be better to ask the parents to wait nearby. 'First aid', i.e. removal of secretions and correct positioning, can be taught when the crisis intervention involving the use of an airway, sucker, oxygen and possibly drug administration is over. Try to find time to listen and talk to them, and find out what happened. Explain the treatment and subsequent investigations, and give them reassurance. As soon as the child is settled and the activity is over, let the mother come in and hold him. It is the best reassurance that they can both have. If the mother is on her own, try to telephone her husband: she will need his support at such a worrying time.

ACUTE EPIGLOTTITIS

One of the most heinous conditions which a child can have is an acutely inflamed epiglottis. Generally the patient starts off with an upper respiratory tract infection and can then very rapidly deteriorate. Croup with marked stridor is often a feature.

The patient can be grey or cyanosed and in an agitated state. Keep the child in the position which seems best, be that in the mother's arms or lying on a trolley. Disturb the child as little as possible. Especially, do not tamper with its neck or even attempt to look into its mouth or the back of the throat. All of these things could compromise the precarious airway. Get senior paediatric and anaesthetic help immediately. Do not leave the child alone or with a junior person for a second. Always have intubation and laryngostomy equipment at hand. Administer a high percentage of humidified oxygen if it can be done without disturbing the child. Gain access to a vein.

Under skilled anaesthesia, it may be possible to intubate the patient. If not, a tracheostomy will be required. The condition should then settle rapidly with antibiotics.

NON-ACCIDENTAL INJURY (NAI)

The problem

So far in this book everything which has been mentioned has been fairly 'clear cut' from the point of view of diagnosis. A patient comes in, you see their injury and believe what they say about it. However, with injuries to children such an approach is not good enough. In a very small group of children, the injuries have been inflicted by adults who are usually their parents. As accident and emergency nurses we therefore have to have a suspicious attitude of the mind when dealing with any injury involving a child. Cases will trickle through and it is up to you to be aware of what can happen so that when an NAI appears it can be spotted. This is yet another example of the importance of routinely asking how an accident occurred and generally chatting with your patients; it pays dividends time and time again. It is only by knowing what the normal result of a given incident looks like that you will ever become suspicious of NAIs.

Child abuse is further complicated by the fact that it does not confine itself to the obvious physical injury such as a cigarette burn. Sexual abuse, in the form of incest or pornography for instance, is far from rare yet is very difficult to latch onto in the confines of an accident and emergency unit.

Psychological neglect or abuse can once again be very subtle in its form and effect on a child, requiring an extremely experienced accident and emergency sister to be able to notice discrepancies. Physical neglect, on the other hand, can be fairly obvious even to those without kids.

Well that is the range of the problem. Frightening isn't it! Now we have to formulate a plan, some guide lines, so that we can firstly discover as many cases as possible and once found act effectively in the best interests of the child.

Recognition

The first stages of recognition have been mentioned already, that is, being suspicious, alert and enquiring. The following pointers are especially important:

- Note the general appearance of the child, whether healthy and well cared for, or ill, undernourished or dirty.
- Try to gather from the expression, actions or words if the child is happy.
- Is he a frequent visitor to the department?
- Has the accident just occurred or has there been a delay of hours or days since the incident?
- Has the 'accident' occurred later in the day than is usual for children's injuries?
- Who has brought the child to the hospital? A friend of the family or relatives?
- Has another person been blamed for the injury?
- Is there more than one injury, which is perhaps of more than one type?
- Can you see injuries (e.g. bruises) of different ages?
- Does the history sound plausible and fit with the injury?
- Is there any previous history of NAI?

Finally, a great danger must be mentioned: jumping to conclusions. Parents may be filthy and aggressive, the children thin and covered with bruises, but that does not mean the parents do not love them very much and do their best for them. Parents can also be well dressed and educated, the child immaculate, yet the child can be persecuted.

Visual pointers (Fig. 180A, B and C)

Here I wish to show just a few of the more common and easily recognized of the signs so that you have a basis on which to build your knowledge. For further pointers I can suggest no better book than *The Battered Child* by Neil O'Doherty given in the list of

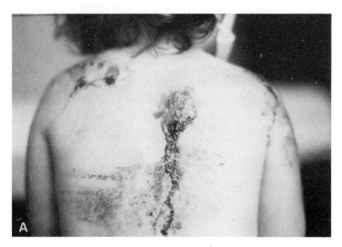

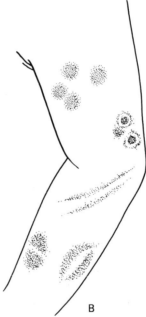

Fig. 180. **A**, *This child was brought into the accident and emergency department three days after injury! Always be alert for cases which may prove to be non-accidental injury and report them.* **B**, *Injury patterns found on the skin, finger marks, cigarette burns, lash marks, and pinch and bite marks.* **C**, *This NAI victim died a few hours later of severe head injuries. A skeletal survey showed fractures of skull, 10 ribs, humerus, radius, ulna, femur and tibia!*

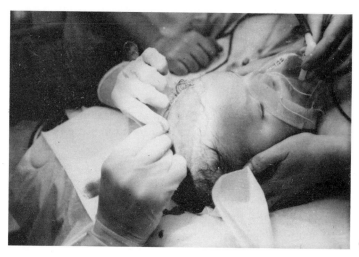

C

Further reading at the end of the chapter. It is really superb and should be read by all accident and emergency nurses.

Action

In all cases of suspected NAI the child should be completely undressed so that a detailed examination can be made. Remember that you, the experienced accident and emergency nurse, may be far more familiar with this sort of problem than the six-month-stay casualty officers, and it is up to you with your suspicions to help them reach the correct diagnosis. Ensure that the undressing and examination, which could be upsetting for the child, are done in the most reassuring and caring way possible. Listen with care to the story given by the parents of how the accident occurred and of the child's health. Try to get an overall picture of the family and any other children. Do not confront the parents with your suspicions. Following examination the doctor will want to list and draw details of all the injuries found. X-rays will be required and often a whole skeletal survey will be done to show up other unsuspected old injuries.

If after examination the doctor has suspicions of NAI, the child should be admitted. Your job has been done and the other experts will take over the child's care and the counselling of the parents.

Our task, therefore, is to draw our suspicions to the attention of others. The paediatricians, the Health Visitor and the Social Services will be alerted according to local hospital policy.

PAEDIATRIC RESUSCITATION

Some aspects of paediatric resuscitation differ considerably from what is usual with adults. Let us now mention some of the most important of these:

- Most cardiac arrests are preceded by respiratory difficulty. Let this be a useful warning to you.
- Do not over extend the head when trying to maintain a clear airway since this will have the reverse effect of partially occluding it (Fig. 181).
- When performing ECM, pressure will have to be applied in the mid-sternum rather than the lower third, both to avoid injury to

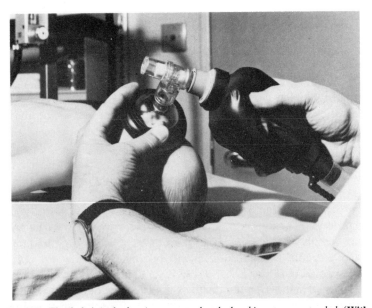

Fig. 181. *The 'baby' Ambu bag in use, note that the head is not over extended.* (**With kind permission of Ambu International**)

the liver and to give more accurate pressure to the higher positioned heart.

- An ECM rate of about 100/min will be required.
- Defibrillation shocks will be power-related to the size of the patient. A rough guide is 20 joules for tiny infants and 75 joules for children.
- The doses of drugs have to be given with far more caution. Sodium bicarbonate is a good example of this, as is adrenaline and calcium chloride. Both adrenaline and atropine may be given via the trachea if great difficulty is experienced in gaining access to a vein. It is essential that a book of paediatric drug doses is referred to so that accurate doses can be worked out depending on the child's weight.
- The major problem associated with paediatric resuscitation, as most of you will have experienced already, will be gaining access to a suitable vein. It can make the most proficient admit defeat.
- Unlike most adults, small infants have very little stored glycogen and can therefore easily become hypoglycaemic; a dextrose infusion is something which the doctor will quite often ask for.
- The size of the endotracheal tube will be variable and a set scale of sizes for ages of children is useful to have around. As a *very* rough working guide look at the size of the child's little finger. An accident and emergency unit must have a full set of sizes constantly available. The smaller tubes will not have any inflatable cuff, any remaining gap being protected by packing the pharynx with moist gauze.

SUDDEN INFANT DEATH SYNDROME (SIDS)

Next I wish to mention cot deaths or sudden infant death syndrome. This condition occurs most commonly before the infant is 8 months old, the exact cause is still not known. Often there has been no associated warning illness, the infant simply being found dead in the cot one morning.

On arrival in the accident and emergency department the child is usually cold, blue or pale, with no signs of life and frequently in rigor mortis. Froth, sometimes bloodstained, can be seen at the nose or mouth and in no way indicate foul play. If the child has been lying on its face the blood will have accumulated in the soft tissues which were dependent, causing an unsightly mottling effect; this is also quite normal.

The parents will be devastated beyond belief, often acting strangely and out of character because of the shock of the death. They will not understand why or how their baby could die and may even feel that they may have done something wrong. Give them all the sympathy and simple support that you can and, if the circumstances are appropriate, brief details of what SIDS is.

When anyone dies unexpectedly in the community like this, the police have to be informed. In fact they will probably have been at the house at the same time as the ambulance. Ensure that the doctor speaks to them immediately so that they realize this is almost certainly SIDS rather than a suspicious death; they can then tread more quietly and compassionately. Let the parents hold their baby, kiss their baby and touch their baby in the privacy of a small room. The Nursing Officer in charge of my accident and emergency department has even gone to the trouble of acquiring delicate, beautiful clothing and shawl to make the experience better for the parents.

Give the parents details in writing, which they can refer to later, of self-help groups which are springing up throughout the country and also offer them an appointment at the Paediatrician's clinic when they are more settled. Finally, ensure that their GP is informed and that immunization reminders are not sent out from the child welfare clinic.

Some final points of general paediatric care are as follows:

• Do your best not to separate the parents from the child. Time and time again I see a mother and child separated on arrival in the department. This lack of contact causes immediate crying. Keep them together, let the clerk take details at the bedside and let the mother help with undressing. If possible, let the mother hold the child on her knee rather than the child being away from her on a bed. Remember that the sight of Mum's face is the only bridge that the child has to the outside 'normal' world, and when you are lost in a terrifying jungle that bridge is a good thing to see and cling onto (Fig. 182).

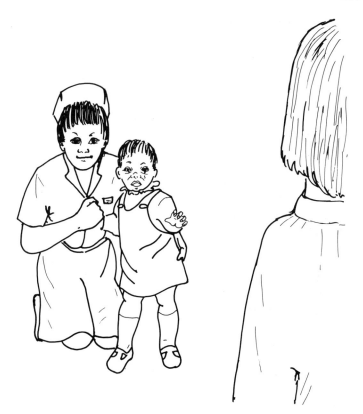

Fig. 182. *Separating mother and child is usually bad.*

- Crouch down to speak to or examine the child. If you are on the same level you will not appear as frightening. Even staying out of the way so that the child is alone behind the screens with Mum while they settle down and get used to the new environment can sometimes be useful with a very nervous child.
- Some children are afraid of people in white coats or of men in general. Try to rectify this with fancy 'play' aprons which nurses can wear or by asking doctors to take off their coats for a while.
- Try to let children get used to a particular nurse or let them be treated all the time by the one they have 'latched onto'.
- As a general rule do not let very junior nurses carry out difficult treatments on tiny children, even mastering the skill of bandaging requires an experienced hand with small patients.

- As part of a routine, try to examine the head for infestation in as many instances as possible. The accident and emergency department is obviously no place for treatment, but we can protect ourselves and other patients from the danger. Inform the parents of what to do or how to get help if the child is going home or inform the ward staff on admission.
- As mentioned in previous chapters, when dealing with children they should be cared for in areas decorated with posters, and a supply of toys should be available.

FURTHER READING

Apley, J. (1979) *Paediatrics*, 2nd edn. London: Baillière Tindall.

Dingwall, R. (1983) Detecting child abuse (in accident departments). *Nursing Times*, 79 (15 June), 66–69.

Illingworth, C.M. (1982) *The diagnosis and primary care of accidents and emergencies in children*, 2nd edn. Oxford: Blackwell.

Jones, D.N. et al (1982) *Understanding child abuse*. London: Hodder & Stoughton.

O'Doherty, N. (1982) *The battered child*. London: Baillière Tindall.

Valman, H.B. (1979) *Accident and emergency paediatrics*. Oxford: Blackwell.

16   The elderly patient

The elderly are among, if not the most neglected of groups in our health service today. From purely an accident and emergency point of view, we can care for them as well as any other group of patients. However, the crunch comes when we try to get them admitted to hospital. It is here that departments the length and breadth of the country encounter problems.

The basic problem is that not enough money is provided for the care of the elderly. This takes effect in two ways. Firstly in the community where there is little in the way of sheltered accommodation for those who are not able to look after themselves properly but are not sick or not sick enough to merit a hospital bed, and secondly in hospital where there are not enough beds for those who are sick.

To compensate for the basic problem is a strategy that the elderly should be able to stay in the community and maintain their independence for as long as possible. This is in essence a fine idea which I am wholeheartedly behind. However, it is sadly abused and is used by some as a reason for turning patients away from hospital. It is here that the accident and emergency department comes into the picture. We are at the front of the 'firing line' so to speak, having to do the 'dirty work' of others in turning away those who are unable to look after themselves adequately (Fig. 183). Of course, it is the doctors of the medical firm who come down to see the patients and say *no*, but it is still the accident and emergency nurses who in reality send the patient off home again to a community nursing service, who with the best will in the world, cannot hope to cope adequately.

In many cultures the elderly remain the head of the family group until their death, their knowledge and experience is greatly acknowledged and they are cared for by the family when they become unable to look after themselves. This is not the case in Great Britain. Here the trend is for sons or daughters to marry and then move away to start their own lives, only occasionally referring to their parents for information or advice. The parents can become infirm as they become elderly and they are often on their own.

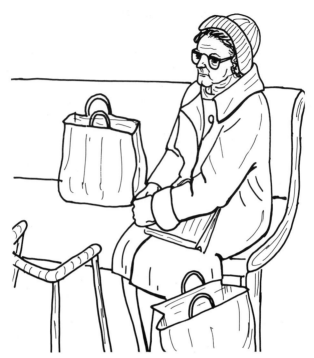

Fig. 183. *The accident and emergency staff still have the 'dirty' job of turning the elderly away.*

This sets the stage for one of the most tragic aspects of life in our society.

Because of this majority way of life it is unfair to expect settled married couples to alter their way of living to accommodate an elderly infirm parent. This is especially true when it would or could cause excessive tensions because of:

- Housing problems — shortage of space, moving children into one room.
- Work problems — giving up a job to look after Mum or Dad
- Health problems — e.g. wife has a bad back and has difficulty in lifting or husband is mentally unstable
- Marriage problems — having to care for an elderly relative could destroy an ailing relationship and be 'the straw which breaks the camel's back'

- Personality problems — not all elderly folk are 'sweetness and light'

So be very wary of criticizing relatives for not inviting their mothers and fathers to live with them; in many instances it is totally unrealistic for us to expect them to do it, although a blessing when they do. At times you can see the weariness in a daughter's eyes. She is at her wit's end after caring valiantly for her mother for some time 'through thick and thin', often with piteously little help. These people look old beyond their years and have been little more than nurses and housemaids often for years. These are the people that we on accident and emergency should identify and help.

You will have realized that, especially with the elderly, we need to know a great deal about the patient's background before we can make an educated decision as to where best to send the patient after treatment. This is far more the case than with a road accident victim, for instance. The only way to do it is to sit down with them and also their relatives, and have a chat (Fig. 184). This must be

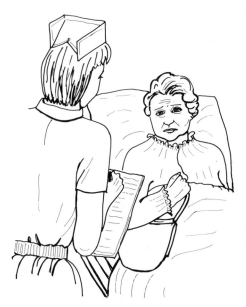

Fig. 184. *When assessing an elderly patient you need to sit down with them and appear to have all the time in the world.*

done even if you are very busy. If it has to be put off temporarily then the patients should be kept in the department until you have assessed them. Never let your patients go home without knowing their circumstances. The accident and emergency department is no place for writing reams of information on a patient's background, but a whole host of information can be put into a form such as that shown in Fig. 4 in Chapter 1. It only takes a few minutes to fill in.

HYPOTHERMIA IN THE ELDERLY

In most units, the common presentation of hypothermia is an elderly patient and this condition is most commonly seen during the winter months. The patient, who is usually female and living on her own, has had an acute episode (a fall or sudden illness) which has immobilized her on the floor in her house, often in a cold bedroom. After a varying length of time someone has become suspicious and the patient has then been discovered, frequently in a very sorry state.

Take the patient's temperature in the rectum using a low-reading thermometer. Leave it in for a substantial time to be sure of the result. A temperature of about 35°C should arouse your suspicions but I do not think, from the nursing point of view, that any exact temperature should be mentioned as drawing the line between normality and hypothermia. The state of hypothermia in such instances, although deadly in itself, is only one aspect which is to be considered. The patient is often dehydrated, undernourished and confused. She may also have complex social problems.

Care in the accident and emergency department

The patient should be warmed gradually. This entails placing the trolley in a warm part of the department. The patient's clothing will have to be removed; it will often be sodden with urine and faeces. The fact that you find her in this state will upset any patient who in earlier years had been very particular about personal hygiene. Some simply break down crying or cling tightly to the clothes so that you cannot see the state that they are in. However, with tact the patient can be comforted; any repulsion you may have must not show. After the patient has been cleaned up, cover her with a polythene 'space blanket' which will retain most of the body heat and place an ordinary blanket on top of this. Alternatively, engulf her with two or three warm blankets. Warm drinks will also be useful, but remember that the mouth may require toilet first.

If the doctor requires an ECG, ensure that this is done before the space blanket is applied, otherwise the trace obtained will be very strange.

Hearing difficulty. Never presume that all old people are deaf. It is very easy to do and I have made this mistake myself in the past. Speak to them in a normal manner and adjust your voice if necessary. I will never forget a very firm rebuke that I received from one very old lady 'Young man, you don't have to shout at me; I'm not deaf. I can hear as well, if not better than you!' If your patient does have difficulty in hearing, first think of the obvious. Does she have a hearing aid and if so, is it adjusted correctly. Often, their deafness has been slow in onset and no hearing aid has been obtained. Never shout at your patient, face her, speak clearly and let her see your lips. Do not try to exaggerate the lip movements. Sometimes a relative may be able to make her understand when you cannot. Give it a try anyway. If all else fails, try writing it down or use a form of pointing sign language.

Arrangements for home

When treatment of an elderly patient has been completed we can sometimes run into major difficulties; the older patient cannot be ushered away with as much ease as someone of middle age. The department can easily seem a friendless, bustling, frightening place. Nurses and other staff can so easily seem too busy to care for the individual. A chance comment by you, that you did not think could be heard, could so easily make you seem heartless. So, remember our older folk and be sympathetic to their fussiness, whims and worries. Explain clearly to your patient how you will get her home and that the ambulanceman will come into the waiting room and ask for her. Ensure that the next appointment is definitely made and suggest that you phone her daughter to explain what the doctor has said. Remember that she will get cold if left in a draughty corridor. Remember that if she has had a cup of tea she might want to use the toilet soon afterwards. Remember that you may have given her so many tablets that she cannot remember which are which, and that the writing on the labels may be so small that she will not be able to read it.

VIOLENCE TOWARDS THE ELDERLY

Finally, I wish to mention violence towards old people. This is often inflicted by close relatives, the so-called 'granny bashing'. In many instances it is carried out by otherwise perfectly reasonable relatives who have been caring for their aged Mum or Dad, or both, for many years. They are often 'at the end of their tether' because of the stress and have frequently had very little help from society.

If you are suspicious that injuries may stem from such a cause, then either the social services and a health visitor will have to be involved to see if they can get to the bottom of the problem, or, if you are very concerned for the immediate safety of the elderly person, you will have to arrange for her to be admitted to hospital.

All in all, it is a very difficult situation. The enormity of this problem is only now starting to show throughout the country.

THE PATIENT WHO IS BROUGHT IN DEAD (BID)

Local arrangements for the reception of patients who are BID or who die in the department will differ considerably. In some areas patients brought in dead are taken directly to the mortuary. In others the patient comes into the department. Whatever system prevails, from our point of view the following items have to be attended to:

1. The body must be inspected by a doctor to certify that death has occurred. Mistakes do happen. If the doctor is in any doubt, the patient must be brought into the department.
2. Relatives must be informed and handled with tact and sympathy.
3. If the body is in the department, it must be segregated with adequate screening.
4. The body must be labelled in whatever way is agreed by the hospital.
5. No 'last offices' are to be performed, simply a 'tidy up'.

6. The patient's clothing and property are to be checked and documented by two nurses.
7. It is essential that the patient is removed rapidly from the department so that valuable admission space is not blocked.

How to 'tell the relatives'

Experienced accident and emergency nurses are ideally suited to the task of informing relatives of the death of their loved ones. It is a horrible job, no one denies that. However, the reward of knowing that you have done it skilfully cannot be surpassed. It will become a natural extension of your patient care, the final service which you can do. In accident and emergency nursing, it is sometimes the only service to be done for the patient. Some may ask if it is not the doctor's job: the answer is probably yes, but only because of tradition. Our training and everyday work bring us into far closer contact with and understanding of patients and their relatives. Even technical details, if required, can be more easily understood in a nurse's familiar language. The subject of talking about death is so delicate and individual that it will take you a long time before you are fully proficient.

To start, go in with an experienced charge nurse or sister and see how he or she approaches the task with different types of people. Compare what they do with my ideas and try to sort out in your mind what your approach would have been.

It is a help to go into the room prepared, knowing as much as possible about the people. The nurse's first tool is a quiet comfortable room near the activity of the department and kitchen. It should have easy chairs, a table, ashtrays and paper tissues; a telephone is also useful. Before entering the room find out the history of how the 'incident' occurred from the ambulance men. Ask how the relatives have reacted and what they know already. For example, do they have a fair idea that the patient is dead or are they quite ignorant of the seriousness of the situation. Gather as many details of the patient as you can beforehand (e.g. name, age, address, religion, family doctor) as this avoids having to ask questions at awkward times. If the patient is a Catholic ask for the services of a priest at once. Lastly be 100 per cent sure that you are speaking to the correct relatives about the correct patient!

The approach. It is pointless trying to get a compassionate message over when you are standing up and distant from the person concerned (Fig. 185). This very position will impart coldness. Ideally, you should be sitting or crouching at the same level as the person you are talking to, possibly with an arm round the shoulders or holding a hand (Fig. 185). This will impart warmth and feeling. Introduce yourself and give a brief greeting. Then, depending on the reactions of the relatives, either say at once what has happened or lead into it more slowly. If nice words fail you, even 'I'm sorry, he's passed away', if said softly with kindness and compassion, will be satisfactory.

After the initial telling comes the reactions, which can vary enormously: sobbing, crying, staring, talking, fighting, fainting or screaming. Some shout out, pleading for the return of the patient. Some relatives just believe you and sit quietly. This is where we see the very best or worst of people. From then on they may act completely out of character. When dealing with situations like this you will need every ounce of tact that you have ever learned.

The worst part of your job is now over, so allow periods of quiet and thought. Incessant chatter is very bad; rather, attempts should be made to lead the relatives into talking about their own thoughts. Listen to what they have to say over a cup of tea or coffee. Find out if the relatives are of a 'religious' inclination and adjust your conversation accordingly. Perhaps you can lead the conversation to the past 'good times'. At a suitable stage find out names and telephone numbers of other relatives or friends who could provide transport home. Never allow the relatives to blame themselves for what has happened; put over positive ideas. Use approaches such as 'No one could have done anything' or 'You did all that anyone could have done'.

It is important that learners are also given the opportunity of going in with you when you talk to relatives, indeed, they are often of considerable help showing great natural compassion. It is only by this 'apprenticeship' that they will see this as one of their roles and become conversant with meeting death head on. It is not uncommon for the learners to be moved to tears by the situation and it is also not a bad thing. Talking it through afterwards with the sister puts the whole experience into perspective and we all come away better nurses. Never try to prevent relatives from

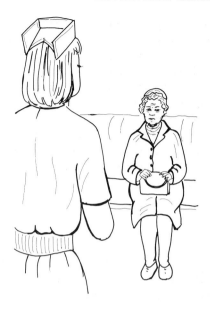

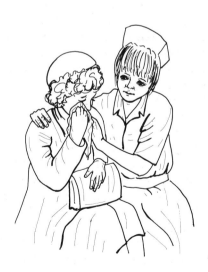

Fig. 185. *Distance from the relatives will impart coolness; closeness will impart warmth and feeling.*

viewing the patient's body. Some will not want to, but those who do should be given every encouragement. Hugging, holding hands, kissing or just crying over the body all help the relatives to come to terms with the fact of death and with their grief.

Before a 'viewing' always ensure that the patient is nicely presented. Clean the face, brush the hair, remove secretions from the nose and mouth; ensure that the pillow is spotless and does not have the Area Health Authority name branded on it for all to see. Fold the blankets with care to hide the mechanisms of the trolley, its lack of paint or splashings of blood. The choice of room is obviously limited, but with care even certain fluorescent lights can be switched off to give a shaded peaceful view. And finally, when they are together allow them to spend some time if they want to, rather than expecting them to just have a quick look.

Allow a reasonable time, about 20 minutes, for the news and talking. Too short or too long a time both have unsettling effects on the relatives. Ensure that transport home is arranged and that someone is available at home for comfort; the initial trauma of entering an empty house can be terrifying. Be aware that, throughout the encounter, the most senior relative present is not always the most sensible or able. A younger son or daughter may be the one who 'rallies' best and should be given the leadership of the family.

More distant relatives will occasionally approach you asking for sleeping tablets or tranquillizers for the bereaved person. I have yet to see a tablet which helps sorrow. Grief is something which has to be felt before it will go away, no matter how unpleasant it is for the onlooker. Supporting the person at home and the effects of time itself offer the surest, smoothest road back to normality. Unless bereavement coincides with a disease drugs should not be advised.

Finally, assistance and advice should be given to the relatives about:

1. A possible post mortem
2. The death certificate
3. Release of the body
4. Undertakers
5. Cash and valuables
6. Clothing

The information given will vary from hospital to hospital depending on local routines.

FURTHER READING

Jones, W.H. & Buttery, N. (1981) Sudden death, survivors' perception of their emergency department experience. *American Journal of Emergency Nursing.* January/February 1981.

17 The ambulance service and its equipment; flying squads

In the accident and emergency unit we are but a link in a long chain, from accident to recovery (Fig. 186). The second link in the chain is the ambulance service. If the link is strong and joined firmly to the remainder of the chain, great things can be accomplished.

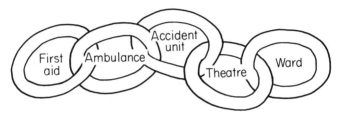

Fig. 186. *The chain of patient care.*

THE AMBULANCE SERVICE

A good liaison with the ambulance service is essential for the smooth running of any accident service. The ambulance crew must be included far more in what happens to a patient after arrival in the department. It is only by being on friendly terms with the crew, answering their questions, letting them work alongside us and having friendly discussions that their standards will ever be considerably and lastingly improved.

Just as ambulance personnel have much to learn from us, we also have much to learn from them. I think that every new staff nurse in an accident and emergency department should spend a week with the ambulance service: seeing and using ambulance equipment, understanding the service's organizational difficulties; finding out what it's like to be out on one's own without a doctor. It would be an eye-opener.

Ambulance men and women in many parts of the country are extending their skills to include insertion of intravenous infusions,

intubation, reading a cardiac monitor, defibrillation and administration of drugs on medical advice. This is a move to the American
paramedical model. Ambulance personnel are trained by doctors
and nurses and are accountable to the employing authority.

In this book all I can do effectively is give a brief outline of the
equipment which some vehicles carry and give a brief insight into
the service's problems. But remember that each authority has its
own rules and standards. Although plans are afoot for eventual
standardization of skills, equipment and methods throughout the
country, these are still in their infancy.

Some of the service's difficulties

1. In hospital, even if we are short-staffed we can get help in an
   emergency, be it extra staff from the wards, a cardiac arrest
   team or a passing houseman. The ambulance crew are truly
   on their own, with no chance of skilled assistance. This
   situation is worsened during the journey to hospital because
   obviously one person must drive. This lack of assistance must
   be reflected in the amount and quality of the aid which they
   can give.
2. The average ambulance is not ideally equipped. Efficient
   electric suction machines have only become commonplace in
   the last few years and are far from universal. If a doctor
   happens to pass the scene of the accident, he will not be able
   to set up an infusion, intubate or give drugs, because none
   exist. Shown in Fig. 187 is the inside of a modern emergency
   ambulance. Compared with many of its counterparts on the
   Continent the equipment is primitive.
3. The design of ambulances leaves much to be desired. The
   ride is uncomfortable for the patient and swaying makes
   performing tasks difficult for the ambulance man. Lighting is
   poor compared to that in an accident and emergency unit.
   The attendant can get to only one side of the patient. There is
   little room at the patient's head for efficient resuscitation,
   although this can be advantageous in a fast ride, wedging
   yourself against the bulkhead.
4. Relatives can be watching everything which is done, expecting something to be done even if the position is hopeless. If
   out of humanity the ambulance crew do nothing they have the
   fear of recriminations.

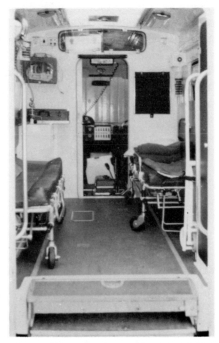

Fig. 187. *The inside of an emergency ambulance.*

5. Frequently the ambulance crew have to look after more than one, often seriously ill, patient. Patients and relatives can also be aggressive, drunk or violent yet the crew are alone.
6. The ambulance crew's knowledge is less than that of doctors and nurses, yet they still have to cope with the most serious conditions without any help.

How to help

If the ambulance crew have a direct radio link with the hospital accident and emergency unit, ensure fast efficient, decisive answers to any queries. If the crew have a serious casualty you should be outside, ready to meet them at the door. The moving of the patient from the ambulance to the accident and emergency department will occupy both of the crew and you will be required to continue resuscitation. The crew are a valuable source of information about the patient; ask a senior nurse to take all the details which will be needed. Even with routine patients a definite 'handing over' of care to the nurses must exist to eliminate the risk of a patient just being left. If the ambulance crew have a little time to spare, let them stay to see the patient undressed and all injuries discovered. Discuss with them what has been done and the likely outcome of the case. Later, if the same crew pass through again, show them any radiographs, ECGs, etc. to promote their interest and consolidate their knowledge. If they make a mistake, do not just grumble about it, but take the time to teach them the correct method.

More lives will be saved and suffering eased in an area with good communication and liaison between the ambulance service and the accident unit. Where there is this two-way flow of opinion, knowledge and ideas the sky is the limit.

Equipment

We now want to consider some of the more important items of equipment carried in an average emergency ambulance.

The stretcher. The stretcher (Fig. 188) is shown raised and with a head-down tilt for an unconscious patient. It is soft and not an ideal surface for external cardiac massage. It is capable of extending to waist height; sides are provided but are only small and relatively inefficient.

Canvas carrying sheet. The canvas (Fig. 189) is strong and durable, invaluable for extracting patients from 'tight' spots. It can be made rigid with poles and spreaders when out in the open. The patient is lifted initially onto the canvas and stays on this all the time. Canvases are interchangeable with others at the hospital.

Scoop stretcher. The scoop (Fig. 190) is a very clever device. Half the scoop stretcher slides under the patient on either side. The two halves are then fixed together and the patient can be lifted with the minimum of movement.

Vacuum mattress (see Fig. 125). The mattress is filled with small granules. The patient is laid on the mattress and it is moulded round

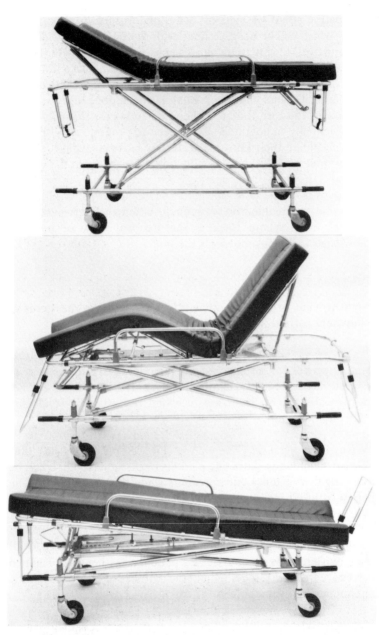

Fig. 188. *An ambulance stretcher in various positions.* (With kind permission of F.W. Equipment Co. Ltd)

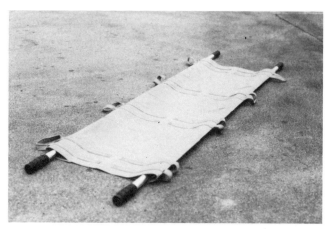

Fig. 189. *A canvas carrying sheet. It can be made rigid with poles and spreader.*

the body. Air is then removed and it becomes as rigid as a board. I have seen a patient with a fractured spine transported over very rough ground very comfortably with this device and it is also used extensively in helicopter transport.

Inflatable splints. Inflatable splints are especially good for use with fractures of the lower leg, but must be of a sensible design with a

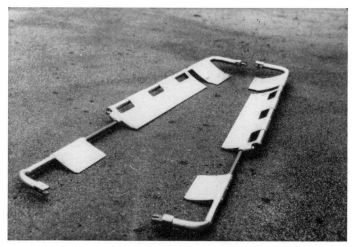

Fig. 190. *The scoop stretcher.*

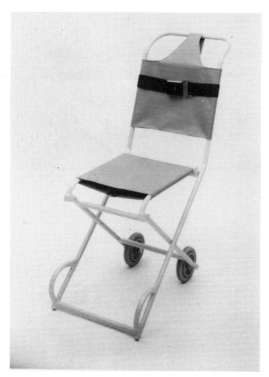

Fig. 191. *The ambulance wheelchair.* (**With kind permission of F.W. Equipment Co. Ltd**)

zip all the way down to the toes, otherwise it will be difficult to put them on painlessly. Some designs are available for use on a fractured wrist but have few advantages over an ordinary arm sling.

Ambulance wheelchair. The ambulance chair (Fig. 191) does not look a very exciting piece of equipment, but is one of the most useful. Stretchers just will not fit in many rooms of a house and upstairs is out of the question. It is this sort of tight-fitting situation in which the chair comes into its own.

Minuteman and PneuPac. The Minuteman (Fig. 192A) is a combination of a pressure-cycled respirator, a suction machine and a way of giving oxygen ordinarily by flowmeter. It works from a tiny

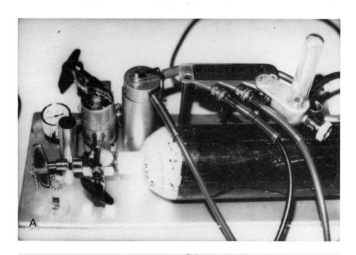

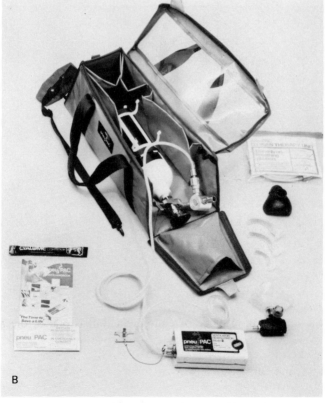

Fig. 192. A, *The Minuteman.* **B,** *The PneuPac respirator.* **(With kind permission of PneuPac Ltd)**

cylinder containing enough oxygen to last for most journeys. It has an extension lead so that it can reach to very confined spaces.

The PneuPac (Fig. 192B) is a robust volume-cycled appliance which does a similar job to the Minuteman. There have been very good reports of it.

Entonox cylinder. Entonox (Fig. 193) consists of 50% oxygen and 50% nitrous oxide. It is a very useful and mobile analgesic which can be used for almost anyone. It takes about two minutes to gain maximum effect. It is used, for example, while splints are being applied at the roadside or when a trapped casualty is being released, but there is no replacement for gentleness.

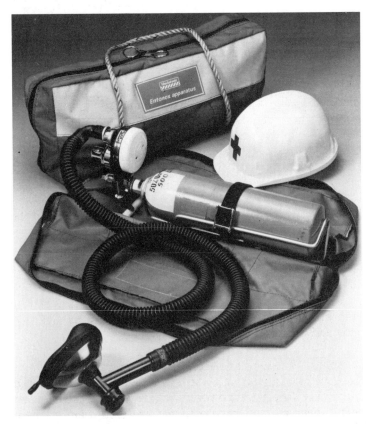

Fig. 193. *The Entonox cylinder.* (**With kind permission of BOC Medishield**)

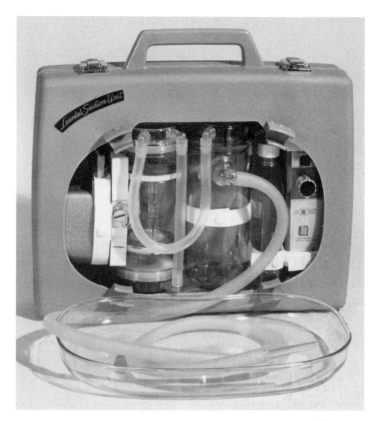

Fig. 194. *The Laerdal suction machine.* (**With kind permission of Vickers Medical**)

Suction. Several suction machines are available for ambulance use. The Laerdal model (Fig. 194) is small, portable and efficient although it will not stand rough handling. It can work either from the ambulance battery or off its own battery. Small efficient foot-operated suction machines are available and are made by Ambu and Capecraft.

Hand-operated respirators. Respirators such as the Ambu bag (Fig. 195) are in everyday use in our hospitals and need no introduction. One point, however, is that two hands are needed to operate them and the ambulance man therefore cannot do anything else.

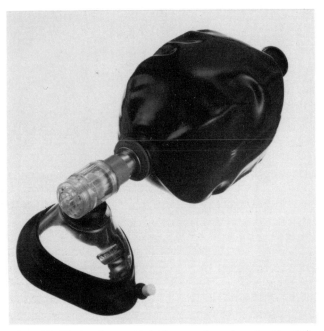

Fig. 195. *The hand-operated Ambu resuscitator (see also* **Fig. 181***).*

Splints. Many types of splints are available, varying from Krahmer wire, which bends to any shape, to rigid plastic covered foam blocks. All have their particular place in the treatment of fractures.

Cervical collar. Cervical collars come in many designs. They are applied to a patient with a neck injury before removal from the scene of the accident. Some like them to be used routinely on unconscious patients 'just in case'. Spinal boards are used in some counties; these are shaped to the body contours and extend from the head to the hips. The head and body are strapped on and the patient is then moved. This minimizes movements.

First-aid kit. A comprehensive first-aid kit is carried, both in small haversacks to take to the scene and in larger containers in the back of the vehicle. Some carry Roehampton burn dressings; these are large sheets of 5 mm foam sterilized and packed. They are placed directly over the extensively burnt area and clipped on; no bandage or extra padding is required.

THE VOLUNTARY AID SOCIETIES

The British Red Cross Society and the St John Ambulance Brigade are two excellent organizations, who among other things train members of the public in first aid. By the time they are in uniform and out doing first-aid duty they should be fairly proficient. Many of them, however, although having the theory, lack much in the way of practical experience of dealing with serious injuries. Members will be able to cope admirably with lacerations or the more common fractures, but may fall down in some respects when dealing with less common conditions such as a major road accident or a difficult airway. The answer of course is education. If first aiders come in with injured patients involve them in what happens. Let them stay with the patients if possible and offer all the advice you can. If they have done well, let them know. The volunteers work hard in their own time to help others and this should be encouraged. It is only by the involvement of such societies and education of the public as a whole that the number of cases of poor or non-existent first aid will drop. I am 100 per cent sure that after you have worked on an accident and emergency unit for six months, you will have said to yourself 'If only someone at the scene knew just a little first aid'!

ACCIDENT FLYING SQUADS

The problem

For years now many in the accident and emergency service have realized that a considerable gap in care occurs between the time of an accident and the patient's arrival at the accident and emergency unit. Let us now look deeper into this gap in our patient's care. For the majority of injuries the presence of doctors, nurses and specialized equipment at the site of an accident is completely unnecessary. The present knowledge and equipment of ambulance men is completely satisfactory for the patient to be given 'ambulance aid' and then taken safely to the nearest accident and emergency unit. The problem, however, arises with the critically injured, the muliple injury, the stove-in chest, the critical airway, the deeply shocked and the trapped limb (I am not mentioning coronary care here as it is a subject on its own). Here the average member of the ambulance crew is out of his depth, in knowledge, experience and equipment. The picture is further darkened if the distance between the accident and the accident and emergency unit is great. In my own district, for instance, everywhere can be reached by road within about 15 minutes; in many areas this figure could be increased three- or fourfold. The result must be more fatalities and suffering.

The answers

I will now describe some methods which are available, or could be available in the future.

The Heidelberg system. Since the early 1950s Professor Gogler, formerly of Heidelberg, has been interested in such schemes, and initiated the present scheme run at the University Surgical Clinic, Heidelberg, West Germany. It attacks the problem in two ways. Firstly, the ambulances are superbly equipped. They have two types, those for everyday 'run-about' use and some which are especially for accidents. The amount of equipment in the accident ambulances is outstanding—all that anyone could wish for. Secondly, there is an emergency car, once again loaded with resuscitation equipment.

A team of enthusiastic surgeons, at registrar level and above, runs the scheme, taking it in turn to be on call. When 'bleeped' the doctor goes to the car which is outside the accident and emergency unit or outside his house and makes his way as quickly as possible to the scene of the accident. The service is used on average twice in 24 hours, the doctor often arriving before the ambulance. If the ambulance arrives first, many of the ambulance crew are able to set up intravenous infusions and to intubate until the doctor arrives. The doctor will travel back to the accident and emergency department with the patient in the amubulance while the police follow on with the emergency car.

Anyone can call the doctor out but with the majority of cases it is the police who call when they first hear of the accident. The staff agreed with me that with this system they were often called to someone who did not need the skills of a doctor, but they were all happy to do this rather than to be selective and 'miss' occasionally.

The immediate 'urgency' of the reception of an accident victim, which is seen so much in the UK, just did not occur. The majority of cases of major trauma arriving at the unit had had their airways cleared or intubated and were already being infused. Shocked patients had already had blood samples taken at the roadside and most major injuries had already been diagnosed.

My overall impression of the medical care was of enthusiasm and learning. Nurses, however, played no part in the scheme whatsoever—a sad reflection.

A separate vehicle is set aside for transfer of neonates in incubators over large distances.

A helicopter ambulance service (Fig. 196) is also used extensively in the area. The helicopters are owned by individual hospital complexes or the army. Bringing patients in from the motorways or nearby hospitals, the helicopters cut down travelling time considerably. Two to three times a week is the usual frequency of this service to the accident and emergency unit. Once they are in the air, little can be done for the patient because the doctor is strapped to a seat at the patient's head; because of this a

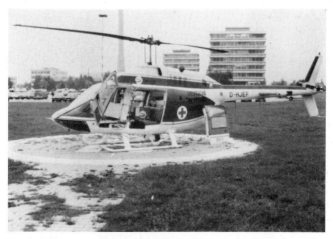

Fig. 196. *A helicopter on the landing pad at Heidelberg. It had just brought in a road traffic accident victim.*

considerable amount of work has to be done to the patient before take-off so that his condition will be reasonably stable in flight.

General practitioner systems. Enthusiastic general practitioners in several parts of the country, notably Easton in Yorkshire, also provide a first-class service. The doctors' private cars are well stocked with resuscitation equipment and other items required at the scene of an accident. The doctors are contacted by radio, bleep or telephone and make their way to the scene of the accident. The ambulance is usually the first to arrive, calling on the services of the doctor if required. The system obviously has tremendous advantages where the accident and emergency unit is a very long distance from the site of the accident, since the general practitioner can be there literally within minutes, whereas a hospital-based team would take too long.

The emergency car system. A shining example of this was the service once organized by Dr Little at Chester. A powerful estate car had been custom-built to carry all the necessary resuscitation equipment and a team of doctors to the scene of an accident (Fig. 197). The equipment was effectively packed into foam-cushioned cases and was quite the most comprehensive that I had ever seen.

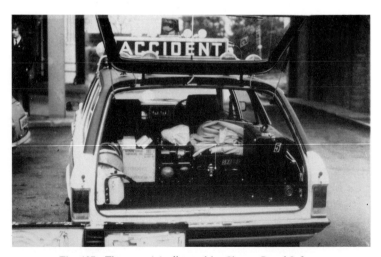

Fig. 197. *The car originally used by Chester Royal Infirmary.*

The car, which was driven by ambulance personnel, was stationed at the accident and emergency unit; it had first-class radio communications and accident equipment.

The well-equipped ambulance. Yet another variation of the flying squad principle is the conversion of an ambulance into what could be termed a 'mobile resuscitation room'. A good example of this is seen at Preston, designed by Mr Hall. The patient is placed on a centrally mounted trolley with the vast amount of equipment scattered around (Fig. 198). The ambulance is based centrally and called out mainly by the attending ambulance if found necessary.

The majority system. The system used by most is to have a collection of resuscitation equipment kept on the accident and emergency unit and a list of personnel 'on call' to go out in an emergency. Transportation is performed by either the police or

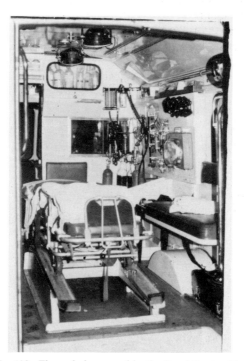

Fig. 198. *The ambulance used by the Royal Preston Hospital.*

the ambulance service. The major drawback here is the time taken for the police or ambulance to get to the hospital to collect the squad and to load the equipment. The majority system therefore is not the best system.

Which is best? Who can say? Distances, personalities, availability and many other factors vary so much from place to place that choice is a very personal matter. My own opinion is that the Heidelberg system just has the lead on the emergency car system because for every severe accident a lavishly equipped ambulance attends the scene with personnel in it who can give an intravenous infusion and intubate if they arrive before the doctor.

The future

What of the future? All the above, in the long term, can be thought of only as temporarily filling a gap until the ambulance staff receive training far in excess of anything so far envisaged. Such a change will take many years, but it is already under way in that the Association of Emergency Medical Technicians (AEMT) is giving training on a local voluntary basis. The other possibility is that experienced accident and emergency nurses will eventually drift into this 'paramedic' situation, more speedily and ably bridging the gap than would ambulance personnel.

Take-out equipment

Many varieties of container exist for hospitals to take out their equipment to an incident. Some I have seen are very poor in design, others quite good. But I have never seen one which is perfect in every respect. Below are listed some of the main points in design which have to be fulfilled if the container is to be ideal.

1. Units must be compact.
2. Each unit must contain all the basic equipment for resuscitation.
3. It should be possible to see every item when the unit is opened, i.e. nothing underneath something else.
4. Everything must be easily removed.
5. Cases must be robust, light and waterproof.
6. They must contain a source of light.

The nurse in the flying squad

This brief section is meant as a rough guide for those nurses who have never been called out with a flying squad, so that they will know what to expect and therefore be able to react more efficiently.

Firstly, confirm with your nursing officer that you are adequately insured. Protect yourself by wearing the protective clothing provided by the hospital; this can seem strange when you first put it on in our sheltered hospital environment. But outside conditions can be extremely rough in the cold and wet. I have often shivered at the roadside, even when I have had several layers on.

Before you leave gather as much detail of the event as you can from the ambulance service. This step is especially important if your take-out 'kit' is comparatively small. You do not want to look foolish at the roadside because an important piece of equipment is missing (Fig. 199).

One of your major duties is to ensure that all equipment is topped up, in working order, easily accessible and that you are *familiar* with it.

On the journey to the scene of the accident be wedged firmly into your seat and be able to brace yourself to prevent being thrown about while the vehicle is cornering. Use the time effectively looking quickly through the equipment, and running a drip through so that it is ready to be 'hooked up' as soon as you arrive. Transfer i.v. cannulae, swabs and strapping to your pocket so that even if you are separated from your kit you are still effective: a drip is almost always required.

Do not presume that the doctor will be a dynamic leader. You may be the one who has more experience of handling casualties outside the hospital setting and the doctor may only have been in the accident and emergency department for a short time. Therefore consider the possibility that you may have to organize the care at the scene.

Find out how many casualties there are. In the ordinary call-out situation there will usually be only one or possibly two. Have a look at all the casualties and decide which deserves priority in care. Do not be misled by others at the scene of the accident who may have misjudged the priorities. It is all too easy to be drawn to the bloodiest or nearest patient while another quietly slips away into unconsciousness or death.

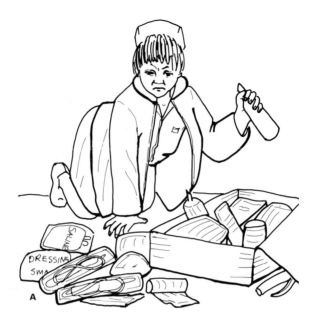

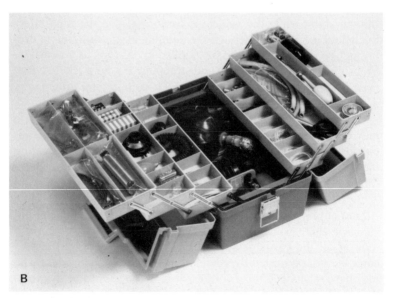

Fig. 199. *A kit where everything can be easily seen is essential.* (**B, with kind permission of Ambu International**)

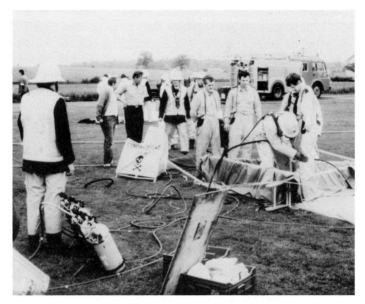

Fig. 200. *Fire brigade decontamination area.*

In many instances you will find that it can be difficult to get near the patient, the emergency services being like a 'rugby scrum' round the victim. However, when you have been called out a few times you will gain experience and tact in 'tackling'!

If conscious, the patient will obviously be very relieved to see you so *look* confident even if you are terrified. Talk, hold his hand and reassure: it all helps. As with any patient in the hospital setting, work through the essentials as soon as you arrive: pulse, breathing, airway, circulation, pneumothorax, haemorrhage.

Policemen make excellent 'drip' stands, so do not get weighed down unnecessarily yourself. Holding drip bottles is also a useful ploy to settle someone who is panicking. Keep an eye on your 'kit' for two reasons: firstly it is very easy for parts of it to be mixed up with that of various ambulances attending the scene or simply lost under debris, and secondly it is not unknown for people to trample all over it in their desire to assist the trapped victim.

Now and then you will be called out to someone who strictly does not need the specialized skills of a flying squad. You will quickly recognize this because of your superior knowledge and experience but it can be far more difficult for other emergency personnel to appreciate. Such a situation is a prime example of why it is important to get together with them so that both sides have a better understanding. Road traffic accidents in which people are trapped are highly charged situations. On occasions you must be prepared for 'masterly inactivity' even though this may seem difficult. Your outward show of calm and experience will have a tremendous sedative effect on those present.

THE CARE OF A PATIENT FOLLOWING A CHEMICAL SPILLAGE

Just over twelve hours after a visit I made to a local fire brigade to see how they cope with a chemical spillage, a very serious accident occurred on a motorway just a few miles from my hospital. Two tankers were involved, one containing petrol and the other ethanol. The driver of one of the vehicles was trapped and a medical team from a hospital nearby was called out to help him. So do not just sit back and skip the next few pages presuming that this cannot happen to you. Fair enough, it may be only once in a lifetime that you will need this information but tomorrow may be that once and if you know a little of what to expect you will be far more able to cope on the day. I consider that the motto to remember in this sort of situation must be 'fools rush in ...'. The only way we can do anything for our patient in such a situation is:

1. If the fire brigade pass the decontaminated patient out to us.
2. If the fire brigade supply us with full protective equipment to approach the lorry cab and then decontaminate us afterwards.

In the first instance we should wait upwind of the incident, the other side of the fire brigade's decontamination area (Fig. 200). The decontamination area is the part of the incident area which has been sectioned off and where they have set up washing down facilities. The patient, if heavily contaminated with a strong substance, must also go through this washing down with cold water and have contaminated clothing removed so that we can safely touch him. Under no circumstances should this routine be broken unless the fire officer on the scene says that the substance is comparatively mild and it is safe for us to go in.

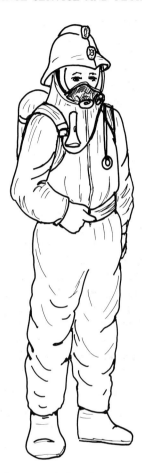

Fig. 201. *Protective clothing for a chemical spillage.*

If the second state exists, i.e. the fire brigade provide us with clothing and go in with us, the following set up is likely to be used (Fig. 201). All permanent members of an accident and emergency department should be familiar with it. Even in remote country districts, tankers pass through on the roads and local casualty departments should be prepared. The local fire brigade will be only too pleased to help if you ask.

Care in the accident and emergency department. Let us now presume that the patient arrives in the department from any source, contaminated with a substance which is thought to be either corrosive, highly irritant or poisonous if it touches our skin. It is unlikely that departments all over the country would be able or willing to provide special protective equipment and clothing for staff. However, a fairly effective protection can be quickly improvised from every day equipment found in most units, i.e. gowns, plastic aprons, rubber gloves, etc.

Further protection can be provided by the plastic anoraks which we use when going out with the flying squad. It must, however, be stressed that all of this is only of limited use, for example, for a patient who has been previously decontaminated by the fire brigade or first aiders, or when a patient has comparatively slight contamination.

In the unit the patient should be laid on the usual accident trolley on top of plastic sheeting with a slight foot-down tilt. The sides of the plastic lap up over cot sides and the end by the feet channel into a large plastic bin. They can then be further washed down with cold water and clothing removed by protected nurses. Water is collected in the bin and clothing can also be placed in there or in plastic bin sacs. A pair of rubber household gloves of the type used by hospital domestics or 'at a push' a couple of pairs of surgeons' gloves will enable most contaminants to be removed. After this the patient can be handled in the normal way. Expert advice from the firm involved with the chemical should by now have been made available to give you further help.

THE CARE OF A PATIENT FOLLOWING A RADIOACTIVE ACCIDENT

Patients contaminated following radioactive accidents can be handled in a basically similar way. But, the advice of a medical physicist should be sought immediately. All departments should have the telephone number of the one who is available for their region. In addition to the precautions already mentioned, the following will have to be thought of:
- If the patient is not seriously ill (I am not talking now of contamination), take him immediately to a cubicle in a comparatively deserted part of the department so that the remainder

of the department is not put out of use. Side doors would be an ideal way in.

- The ambulance should be kept closed until the floors of the unit have been covered with paper or plastic from the ambulance to the cubicle.
- Have a mental picture of radioactive contamination as being like harmful bacteria covering the patient and his clothing like a fine dust, and getting everywhere.
- Keep movement in and out of the cubicle to a minimum, items just being passed in to the staff who are protected, in a similar way to dealing with a chemical spillage.
- Do not throw away any water used in washing the patient down and wait until the physicist arrives with the $\alpha\beta\gamma$-geiger counter.

FURTHER READING

Buckles, E. (1983) A flying squad comes of age. *Nursing Times*, 79:5.
Weeks, L.P.F. (1980) The ambulance service. *Nursing*, 1:14 (June), 592.

Appendix

I. ENDOTRACHEAL INTUBATION

Endotracheal intubation is a 'medical' skill which is becoming increasingly required by senior accident and emergency nurses. It can never be learnt solely from a book because it is essentially a practical skill. This section, however, will give you a grounding on which to build up your skill with frequent practice. It entails positioning a tube between the vocal cords into the trachea. At the end of the standard tubes, in all except the smaller sizes, is an inflatable balloon (like a Foley catheter). This can be inflated and will therefore completely seal off the patient's airway from the danger of aspiration of stomach contents or blood from the mouth.

Positioning of the patient is of prime importance: 'sniffing the air' as it has been classically described (Fig. 202). The patient is placed flat on his back. The head is supported on a small pillow and extended.

The laryngoscope is inserted down the right-hand side of the mouth, pushing the tongue to the left, until the epiglottis is reached (Fig. 203). Quite often at this stage suction will be necessary before anything can be visualized. Two types of laryngoscope blades are in common use: the Magill which has a straight

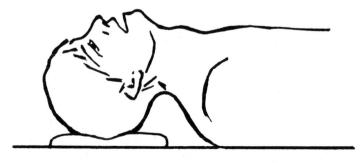

Fig. 202. *The 'sniffing the air' position for intubation.*

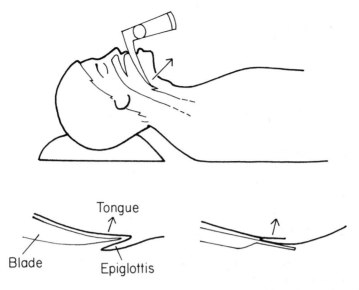

Fig. 203. *The laryngoscope is inserted down the right hand side of the mouth until the epiglottis is reached. The arrow shows the direction of pull which is then put on the blade.* **Inset**, *the epiglottis and the position of the blade.*

blade and the Macintosh whose blade is curved and is the most frequently used. Depending on the type of laryngoscope blade used, the tip of the blade is then placed in the fold between the epiglottis and the base of the tongue (with the Macintosh laryngoscope), then lifted. Alternatively (with the Magill laryngoscope) the blade of the laryngoscope slides over the epiglottis and lifts it directly. Either manoeuvre should now disclose the larynx and vocal cords.

While the larynx is being visualized and the endotracheal tube passed, pressure over the cricoid cartilage (Fig. 204) will help to prevent the escape of stomach contents until intubation is complete. Ensure that the tube is not inserted too far into the trachea. If it does go too far it may enter the right main bronchus causing the left side of the chest not to be inflated. The cuff must next be inflated until you hear the sounds change as it seals to the trachea.

You are now ready to inflate the lungs with oxygen, but it is important to remember that you now have a sealed system and the expiratory valve has to be opened for the escape of used gases.

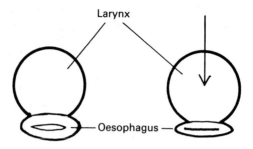

Fig. 204. *Pressure over the cricoid cartilage compresses the oesophagus, helping to prevent inhalation of the stomach contents should vomiting occur.*

If difficulty is encountered either in visualizing the larynx or in introducing the tube, it is best to revert to the airway and bagging rather than make prolonged efforts. It is a mistake to attempt time after time to get the tube down if the airway is otherwise clear. Remember that while you are doing all of this the patient is without oxygen and you are lessening his chances of survival.

One final but nevertheless very important point: there is a tremendous difference between intubating in a theatre with an anaesthetist standing by and a fully prepared patient, and intubating 'out on your own' in an extreme emergency with someone simultaneously doing external cardiac massage. Never attempt intubation until you are confident.

II. VENEPUNCTURE

In the comparative peace and solitude of a ward, getting a needle into a patient's vein can be trying enough. In the frequently tense atmosphere of an accident and emergency unit, with a collapsed patient just in off the street and maybe no doctor in sight, it can be downright tricky. The same principles, however, apply and to try to rush things will frequently end in failure.

First pay attention to the essential preliminaries detailed in Chapter 2. Have an efficient tourniquet round the arm and leave it in place long enough to do its job. Have the elbow fully extended and the arm firmly supported. It may be necessary for two nurses to hold the arm if the patient is very restless. A familiar site should be chosen which, with nurses, will usually be either the antecubital fossa or the radial border of the forearm. Feel first with your fingertips to ensure that it is a vein you can see; superficial arteries and tendons can easily be mistaken. Clean the skin; if visualization is difficult a quick shave may be necessary. Stretch the overlying skin with one hand to help to immobilize the vein.

Insert the needle and cannula almost level with the skin and then gently manoeuvre it into the vein. Check that blood can be withdrawn, then remove the needle. The cannula can then be gently pushed further into the vein before being firmly strapped into position.

Some difficulties

Veins which are very 'obvious', especially in old patients, are often very difficult to enter because they tend to move about under the skin since they have few attachments. It will often be found easier to enter a vein which can be 'felt' rather than seen easily. Vein junctions can sometimes offer more stability.

If the injection site swells, abandon it because it cannot be relied on.

III. DRUGS COMMONLY USED

Adrenaline 1:1000. Commonly used following a cardiac arrest. It helps to convert fine ventricular fibrillation to coarse and asystole to ventricular fibrillation. Isoprenaline has similar properties.

Aminophylline. Relieves bronchial spasm and therefore is used mainly for asthmatics. Commonly 250–500 mg are given intravenously followed by 500 mg added to infusion.

Atropine 600 μg. Speeds up the rate of the heart beat and is therefore used for a patient with bradycardia.

Calcium chloride 10%. Often given following a cardiac arrest to convert asystole to ventricular fibrillation or to aid defibrillation.

Digoxin 500 μg and Ouabain. Similar drugs used to treat atrial fibrillation.

Dopamine hydrochloride (Intropin). This drug will increase cardiac output. 200 mg are added to an infusion in an attempt to raise the patient's blood pressure.

Frusemide (Lasix) 20–25 mg. A very powerful diuretic, commonly used to treat pulmonary oedema.

Hydrocortisone 100 mg. Sometimes used in the treatment of profound shock in massive doses, also for severe asthmatics. Less commonly seen uses include severe head injuries and anaphylactic reactions.

Lignocaine 2% and 20%. Used to prevent or treat some of the arrhythmias seen following a coronary, i.e. ventricular tachycardia and extrasystoles.

Naloxone (Narcan) 0.4 mg. This is used to reverse the actions of the morphine group of drugs. It works within a minute.

Prochlorperazine maleate (Stemetil) 12.5 mg. It is used to prevent vomiting following injections of the morphine group of drugs.

Procyclidine hydrochloride (Kemadrin) 5 mg. Used to combat the extrapyramidal side-effects of certain drugs. It works very quickly stopping occulogyric crises within minutes.

Sodium bicarbonate 8.4%. This drug, which is given by intravenous infusion, is administered after all cases of cardiac arrest. It corrects the acidosis which will be present. See Chapter 1 for dosage regimen.

IV. SUTURE TECHNIQUE

Good suture technique is essentially a practical skill which cannot be learned from a book. However, there follows a brief introduction to the subject, which will guide the new staff nurse during early attempts. The preliminaries to suturing are carried out as mentioned in Chapter 6, pp. 99–101.

Hold the skin gently with the toothed forceps; roughness can damage delicate wounds. The needle must take an equal 'bite' of the skin on either side of the wound (Fig. 205B). For a smooth easy entry the needle should be pressed in, following the shape of its own curve (Fig. 205A). A simple loop design is satisfactory for the majority of the minor wounds seen in an accident and emergency unit. The knot is difficult to master at first but with practice on a piece of spare cloth it will soon become second nature to you. Avoid pulling the knot too tight; the wound edges should be under the minimum tension. Do not be satisfied until the skin edges meet accurately. If one edge of the wound is lower than the other, move the knot over to the other side or try adjusting the levels with toothed forceps.

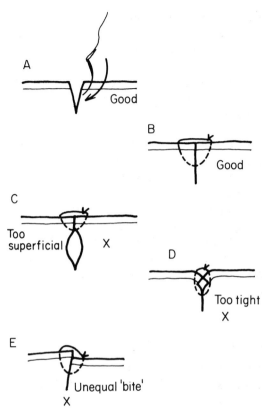

Fig. 205. *Suture technique.* **A**, *push the needle in following its natural curve.* **B**, *an equal bite of skin is taken and only the minimum tension applied.* **C**, *the suture must be deep enough to close the depths of the wound;* **D**, *if it is pulled too tight the edges may invert;* **E**, *if the bite is unequal, a 'step' can occur.*

Some common mistakes

1. Too many sutures inserted. This causes worsening of the scar and hinders the blood supply to the wound edges.
2. Suture inserted too superficially. It should be deep enough to close the depths of the wound (Fig. 205C).
3. Suture pulled too tight. This can invert the wound edges which will delay healing and worsen the scar (Fig. 205D).
4. Sutures too loose.
5. A 'step' in the wound (Fig. 205E).

V. EMERGENCY LARYNGOSTOMY

Most of this section will concern nurses working in outlying hospitals, where it may take many minutes before the doctor arrives to help.

As mentioned previously the accident and emergency department is not the ideal place for a tracheostomy to be performed. The procedure is best done electively at a later date. However, on very rare occasions it is forseeable that a nurse could be in a position in which she is unable to secure the patient's airway with an endotracheal tube and some form of artificial opening is the patient's only hope of survival. The obstruction could be due to oedema, a foreign body or trauma. It is to be stressed that the method described below is *for use by nurses, only when all else has failed*, the patient is moribund and the doctor cannot be obtained immediately.

The patient is positioned on the back with a sandbag under the neck and shoulders. The head should be extended and supported so that it does not twist to one side (Fig. 206).

With the left hand, hold over the thyroid cartilage with the thumb and index finger. With the right hand, locate the cricothyroid membrane and with a scalpel make a small longitudinal incision until the membrane is reached. Make an incision about 2–3 cm long in the membrane and keep this open with tracheal dilators until any form of temporary tube is in place. Bleeding from the incision should be minimal and easily controlled by gentle pressure until the doctor arrives to take over.

Find out when a tracheostomy is about to be performed in your hospital, so that you can go along to observe. It will be an invaluable experience for you. No experience is ever wasted in the field of emergencies.

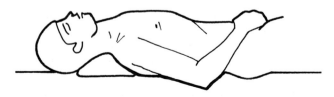

Fig. 206. *The head fully extended for an emergency laryngostomy.*

VI.   ENTONOX

Entonox, which is a 50% mixture of oxygen and nitrous oxide, has been mentioned several times through the book. It is widely used in accident and emergency departments. It can be piped or supplied in large cylinders for use in the departments or very small cylinders which are ideal for the ambulance service. The mixture remains stable unless the temperature drops below approximately $-7°C$. The gas is administered by the patient through a special demand valve. A mask or mouth-piece can be used, but with both an air-tight seal is essential. The patient holds the mask or mouth-piece to the face and breathes in normally. While the patient breathes in, the gas will be delivered. While the patient exhales, the mask or mouth-piece can be left in position. After a few breaths he will start to notice changes, but it will be about two minutes before maximum relief is obtained. Because of this it is important not to start any painful manoeuvre until two minutes after the patient has started to breathe the gas.

Examples of the wide range of uses for Entonox are given below:

1. A trapped patient who is in pain at the scene of a road accident
2. Just about any painful condition as long as the patient is cooperative, while on the way to hospital, e.g. fractured limbs, cardiac pain.
3. While temporarily splinting fractures or undressing patients in the accident and emergency department
4. As an additive to drugs like pethidine while awaiting reduction of fractures
5. Painful dressings
6. Reduction of minor fractures or dislocations
7. Chest injuries

Most children take to Entonox very easily, as long as everything is carefully explained to them first. There are a few, however, who are terrified of a mask over the face. Sometimes this fear can be overcome with the use of the mouth-piece, but great tact is required.

Occasionally after breathing the gas for several minutes, the patient can become restless, start shouting or laughing, and moving arms and legs about. Because of this, your patient should always be lying down, there should be sides on the trolley and someone should be with you in case of mishap. As with all patients in an altered state of consciousness, suction should be at hand in case of vomiting.

FURTHER READING

Michael, D.T.A. & Gordon, A.S. (1980) Oesophageal obturator airway. *British Medical Journal*, 281.

Moore M. (1983) The potential use of Entonox by nurses in A & E departments. *Nursing Times* (6 April).

Index